WHO Health Evidence Network synthesis report 70

Mental health, men and culture: how do sociocultural constructions of masculinities relate to men's mental health help-seeking behaviour in the WHO European Region?

Brendan Gough | Irina Novikova

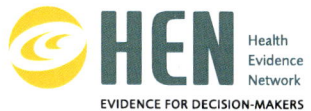
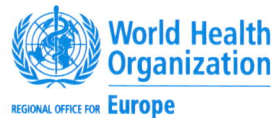

Abstract

Men are less likely than women to seek help for mental health issues and are much more likely to commit suicide. This scoping review examined recent evidence published in English and Russian on the role of socially constructed masculinity norms in men's help-seeking behaviour for mental health issues. The key sociocultural barriers to men's help-seeking pertaining to masculinity norms were identified as self-reliance, difficulty in expressing emotions and self-control. The wider community, societal and cultural challenges to men's help-seeking and well-being were found to include economic insecurity, inequality and limited health- and social-care provision – especially for marginalized groups of men. However, there is also evidence to indicate that men are able to display vulnerability and seek help with trusted people (such as family members, peers and specialists) and within trusted communities. Policy considerations to improve men's help-seeking for mental health issues should include an awareness of the prevailing cultural norms of masculinity in diverse groups of men to provide effective tailored interventions for mental health promotion.

Keywords
MEN, MASCULINITY, MENTAL HEALTH, CULTURE, INEQUALITIES, BEHAVIOUR, GENDER

Address requests about publications of the WHO Regional Office for Europe to:
  Publications
  WHO Regional Office for Europe
  UN City, Marmorvej 51
  DK-2100 Copenhagen Ø, Denmark
Alternatively, complete an online request form for documentation, health information, or for permission to quote or translate, on the Regional Office website (http://www.euro.who.int/pubrequest).

ISSN 2227-4316
ISBN 978 92 890 5513 0

© World Health Organization 2020

Some rights reserved. This work is available under the Creative Commons Attribution-NonCommercial-ShareAlike 3.0 IGO licence (CC BY-NC-SA 3.0 IGO; https://creativecommons.org/licenses/by-nc-sa/3.0/igo).

Under the terms of this licence, you may copy, redistribute and adapt the work for non-commercial purposes, provided the work is appropriately cited, as indicated below. In any use of this work, there should be no suggestion that WHO endorses any specific organization, products or services. The use of the WHO logo is not permitted. If you adapt the work, then you must license your work under the same or equivalent Creative Commons licence. If you create a translation of this work, you should add the following disclaimer along with the suggested citation: "This translation was not created by the World Health Organization (WHO). WHO is not responsible for the content or accuracy of this translation. The original English edition shall be the binding and authentic edition".

Any mediation relating to disputes arising under the licence shall be conducted in accordance with the mediation rules of the World Intellectual Property Organization.

Suggested citation. Gough B, Novikova I. Mental health, men and culture: how do sociocultural constructions of masculinities relate to men's mental health help-seeking behaviour in the WHO European Region? Copenhagen: WHO Regional Office for Europe; 2020 (Health Evidence Network (HEN) synthesis report 70).

Cataloguing-in-Publication (CIP) data. CIP data are available at http://apps.who.int/iris.

Sales, rights and licensing. To purchase WHO publications, see http://apps.who.int/bookorders. To submit requests for commercial use and queries on rights and licensing, see http://www.who.int/about/licensing.

Third-party materials. If you wish to reuse material from this work that is attributed to a third party, such as tables, figures or images, it is your responsibility to determine whether permission is needed for that reuse and to obtain permission from the copyright holder. The risk of claims resulting from infringement of any third-party-owned component in the work rests solely with the user.

General disclaimers. The designations employed and the presentation of the material in this publication do not imply the expression of any opinion whatsoever on the part of WHO concerning the legal status of any country, territory, city or area or of its authorities, or concerning the delimitation of its frontiers or boundaries. Dotted and dashed lines on maps represent approximate border lines for which there may not yet be full agreement.

The mention of specific companies or of certain manufacturers' products does not imply that they are endorsed or recommended by WHO in preference to others of a similar nature that are not mentioned. Errors and omissions excepted, the names of proprietary products are distinguished by initial capital letters.

All reasonable precautions have been taken by WHO to verify the information contained in this publication. However, the published material is being distributed without warranty of any kind, either expressed or implied. The responsibility for the interpretation and use of the material lies with the reader. In no event shall WHO be liable for damages arising from its use.

The named authors alone are responsible for the views expressed in this publication.

Printed in Luxembourg

CONTENTS

▸ Abbreviations iv

▸ Acknowledgements v

▸ Summary vii

▸ 1. Introduction 1
    ▸ 1.1 Background 1
    ▸ 1.2 Methodology 6

▸ 2. Results 7
    ▸ 2.1 Stigma around men's mental health issues 9
    ▸ 2.2 Support tailored to the needs of diverse groups of men 16
    ▸ 2.3 Community-level interventions 19
    ▸ 2.4 Reframing help-seeking within traditional masculinity norms 25
    ▸ 2.5 Rethinking masculinity? 27

▸ 3. Discussion 31
    ▸ 3.1 Strengths and limitations of this review 31
    ▸ 3.2 Beyond masculinities: a need for further research 32
    ▸ 3.3 Policy considerations 34

▸ 4. Conclusions 35

▸ References 36

▸ Annex 1. Search strategy 54

ABBREVIATIONS

CALM	Campaign Against Living Miserably
SDG	Sustainable Development Goal

ACKNOWLEDGEMENTS

This report has been produced with the financial assistance of the Wellcome Trust. The views expressed herein can in no way be taken to reflect the official opinions of the Wellcome Trust.

The authors wish to express their thanks to Lucy Eldred, a postgraduate student at Leeds Beckett University, who helped with English literature search. The authors also acknowledge the valuable feedback received from independent reviewers and panel members who attended the fifth WHO expert group meeting on the cultural contexts of health and well-being in June 2019.

Authors

Brendan Gough
Professor of Social Psychology, School of Social Sciences, Leeds Beckett University, Leeds, United Kingdom

Irina Novikova
Director, Gender Studies Centre and Professor, English Department, University of Latvia, Riga, Latvia

Peer reviewers

Derek M. Griffith
Founder and Director of the Center for Research on Men's Health and Professor of Medicine, Health and Society, Vanderbilt University, Nashville, Tennessee, United States of America

Jeff Hearn
Professor Emeritus, Hanken School of Economics, Finland; Professor of Sociology, University of Huddersfield, Huddersfield, United Kingdom; Senior Professor, Gender Studies, Örebro University, Örebro, Sweden; and Professor Extraordinarius, Institute for Social and Health Studies, University of South Africa, Pretoria, South Africa

Noel Richardson
Director, National Centre for Men's Health, Institute of Technology Carlow, Carlow, Ireland

Editorial team, WHO Regional Office for Europe

Division of Information, Evidence, Research and Innovation

Nils Fietje
Research Officer, Cultural Contexts of Health and Well-being

Shanmugapriya Umachandran
Consultant, Cultural Contexts of Health and Well-being

Division of Noncommunicable Diseases and Promoting Health through the Life-course

Bente Mikkelsen, Director

Dan Chisholm, Programme Manager for Mental Health

Division of Policy and Governance for Health and Well-being

Isabel Yordi Aguirre, Programme Manager

Åsa Nihlén, Technical Officer

Health Evidence Network (HEN) editorial team

Natasha Azzopardi Muscat, Director, Division of Country Health Policies and Systems
Kristina Mauer-Stender, former Acting Director, Division of Information, Evidence, Research and Innovation
Tanja Kuchenmüller, Editor in Chief
Tarang Sharma and Ryoko Takahashi, Series Editors
Tyrone Reden Sy, Managing Editor
Krista Kruja, Consultant
Ashley Craig, Technical Editor

The HEN Secretariat is part of the Division of Country Health Policies and Systems (previously the Division of Information, Evidence, Research and Innovation) at the WHO Regional Office for Europe. HEN synthesis reports are commissioned works that are subjected to international peer review, and the contents are the responsibility of the authors. They do not necessarily reflect the official policies of the Regional Office.

SUMMARY

The issue

Fewer men than women are diagnosed with depression and treated for depression-related disorders and other common mental health problems. This is partly due to the real prevalence of depression being lower in men, which is thought to relate to biological differences between the sexes. However, there is also the compounding challenge of men not seeking help for psychological issues, delaying engagement with therapeutic services until problems deteriorate and being diagnosed with other conditions (e.g. psychosomatic) – that is, depression is hidden or masked by men and is, therefore, underdiagnosed. In addition, health professionals and significant others may not recognize mental health issues in men and may not recommend mental health services when they do. It is important to note that gender norms intersect with wider social change and challenges, including economic hardship, limited mental health service provision, racism and discrimination against marginalized groups of men. Although rates of depression are 50% higher in women than men, suicide rates are approximately three times higher in men than in women and are linked to traditional masculinity factors (e.g. limited emotional disclosure and help-seeking) that are disproportionately experienced by specific groups of men (e.g. gay men, rural men, divorced men, and unemployed or indebted (i.e. who feel they have failed in the traditional breadwinner role) men).

Research to date has focused on the role of masculinities in constraining men's inclination and capacity for emotional communication and service engagement – although a more recent focus has been on the intersection of gender with other identity dimensions (e.g. age, race or sexual orientation), the impact of life events (e.g. bereavement) and the wider social determinants of well-being (e.g. poverty, inequalities or precarious employment). To date, no review has focused on the impact of masculinity norms (and their place within diverse and shifting sociocultural contexts) on men's help-seeking behaviour for mental health problems in the WHO European Region.

The synthesis question

The objective of this report is to answer the question: "How do sociocultural constructions of masculinities relate to men's mental health help-seeking behaviour in the WHO European Region?"

Types of evidence

This report used a scoping review to identify relevant documents in peer-reviewed and grey literature published between 2009 and 2019 in English and Russian. Of the 41 documents identified, 23 were in English and 18 were in Russian. Literature in English comprised diverse methodologies (empirical research, quantitative, qualitative, mixed-methods studies and reviews), whereas literature in Russian primarily comprised opinion pieces and commentaries, with few empirical reports. Additional articles were suggested for inclusion by panel members of a WHO expert group meeting, and contextual information from the fields of men and masculinities, gender studies and men's health with a focus on culture and intersectionality was added by the authors.

Results

The analysis highlighted key themes pertaining to the role of masculinities (and wider community and societal factors) in inhibiting or facilitating men's help-seeking for mental health problems: stigma, support from significant others, community interventions, reframing help-seeking within traditional masculinity norms, and challenging traditional masculinity norms.

Stigma around mental health issues was found to be particularly acute for men, who may lack mental health literacy and fear being judged for exposing vulnerability, especially by other men. Men who closely adhere to traditional masculinity norms (such as self-reliance, difficulty in expressing emotions, independence, dominance and self-control) were less likely to disclose problems to others or seek assistance. Such traditional gender norms are more pronounced in some communities (such as economically deprived environments), leaving little opportunity for many men to show distress or seek help, and this situation may be compounded by limited or culturally inappropriate service provision (e.g. in rural areas) or by particular life events (e.g. retirement, unemployment or divorce). Some men were reported to experience stigma around taking medication for depression and having therapy – although others found that having a clear diagnosis and treatment plan was beneficial because it validated their experiences.

Many men were found to misrecognize depression and, as a consequence, exhibited risk-taking behaviour, such as alcohol and drug abuse, overworking and violence, only seeking help when they experienced a crisis and/or when prompted by significant others, typically women. The influence of traditional masculinity norms on some groups of men was particularly evident in Russian language studies, and within particular institutional and work contexts (e.g. the military, fire brigade and team sports). The importance of intersectional analysis was highlighted by reports that help-seeking may be more challenging for men in specific disadvantaged groups, including refugee and migrant men, black and minority ethnic men, indigenous men, gay and bisexual men, and rural men, where it is linked to local subcultural norms, patterns of prejudice, discrimination and social exclusion. It is clear that men from marginalized communities may avoid accessing therapeutic services that they perceive to be unrepresentative, remote or culturally inappropriate. In addition, traditional masculinity norms can make boys and men experiencing difficult life events, such as bullying, unemployment, illness and bereavement, especially vulnerable to social withdrawal, loneliness and distress. Men are overrepresented in chronically excluded groups, such as homeless people, ex-prisoners and refugees and migrants.

More positively, evidence suggests ways of engaging men in emotional disclosure and help-seeking. Of key importance is to consider the impact of masculinity norms by striking a balance between leveraging dominant ideals to promote engagement and challenging those that constrain men from seeking help. Help-seeking has sometimes been reframed along more masculine lines so that it is perceived to be a strength rather than a weakness (e.g. requiring courage, action and independence) or as a means of regaining valued masculine attributes (e.g. moving from dependence to independence). Similarly, therapeutic services that go beyond just talking to incorporate practical exercises, goal-setting and collaboration were found to be particularly appealing to some men. These approaches fit into the gender-specific approach, as defined in the WHO Gender Responsive Assessment Scale.

Beyond the clinic, online and community interventions offer some promise, as long as men feel safe and trust their peers and mentors, and the approach is informal, collegial and social rather than medical. Such approaches should be tailored to the particular target community by incorporating culturally appropriate representation, language and activities. In addition, interventions that address societal and structural issues (e.g. discrimination, poverty, prejudice and social exclusion) are needed because gender is only one factor in shaping and constraining mental health. Masculinity norms also intersect with issues such as homophobia, racism, job insecurity, unemployment, parenting policies and ineffective service provision to undermine help-seeking and service use for many groups of men – this needs to be recognized by men themselves, communities, and service providers and policy-makers.

Some men who engage in help-seeking and emotional development may start to rethink their masculine identities to incorporate displays of vulnerability and self-care. However, more contemporary forms of masculinity that lack some of the harmful elements of traditional masculinity may only be feasible within certain relationship, community and societal contexts. Therefore, interventions designed to challenge the harmful aspects of traditional masculinities through gender-transformative actions could improve men's health and promote gender equality. The case studies presented in this report offer examples of interventions that have worked well for different groups of men.

Policy considerations

Based on the findings of this scoping review, the main policy considerations to promote and protect men's and boys' mental health in the WHO European Region are to:

- support the mental health needs of the most vulnerable or at-risk groups (refugee and migrant, indigenous, long-term unemployed, sexual and ethnic minority men) by tackling the root causes of disconnection and isolation through addressing the links between gender and homophobia/racism;
- provide resources to enable parents and relevant institutions (e.g. schools or youth centres) to engage boys and young men (particularly those from minority and disadvantaged backgrounds) in critical discussions of gender norms, identities and relations and the links between gender, gender inequality, health and well-being;
- promote collaboration and partnerships between the health sector and community organizations working with diverse groups of men on a range of projects (e.g. cultivating responsible and involved fatherhood, violence prevention, addressing substance abuse);
- educate health- and social-care professionals about how gender influences how men present with mental health problems;
- develop male-friendly initiatives tailored to the values, customs and priorities of those groups of men most in need (such as sports-related activities), and actively engage the target groups in developing such initiatives;
- promote strengths-based approaches to men's mental health that build on positive aspects of traditional masculinity and normalize mental health issues such as depression within diverse communities; and
- engage with health-focused television programmes and websites that provide relevant information and enable men to share their problems with and receive support from experts/peers, and promote online support forums to men in all Member States of the WHO European Region.

1. INTRODUCTION

1.1 Background

The gender and health framework of the WHO European Region comprises two complementary strategies on men's and women's health and well-being. The first component, the Strategy on Women's Health and Well-being in the WHO European Region (resolution EUR/RC66/R8), was adopted in 2016 by the 66th session of the Regional Committee for Europe (1,2). Following this, in September 2017 WHO started a consultation with experts in a range of fields and disciplines related to gender and men's health, from civil society and from Member States of the Region with the aim of developing a WHO strategy and report on using gender approaches to improve the health and well-being of men and boys in the Region. Preparation of the report involved a consultation process aimed to increase the understanding of how men's health needs, men's health-seeking behaviour and the responses of health services and systems are influenced by gender norms, levels of gender equality and the wider social determinants of health. The Strategy on the Health and Well-being of Men in the WHO European Region (resolution EUR/RC68/R4) was adopted by Member States at the 68th session of the Regional Committee for Europe in September 2018 (3,4), and a report of the recommendations of the Strategy was launched during the same session (5). The Strategy was built on the guiding principles of the 2030 Agenda for Sustainable Development (6) and Health 2020 (7) and on the interconnected nature of the Sustainable Development Goals (SDGs) (8), notably SDG 3 (good health and well-being) and SDG 5 (gender equality). During development of the Strategy, the impact of masculinity norms (and their intersection with diverse sociocultural contexts) on mental health help-seeking in the WHO European Region was identified as a key area for further research.

Men's mental health is a key area for improvement within population health, within the Region and globally. An increased understanding of why and how men seek help for mental health issues is vital for improving these outcomes and the wider outcomes beyond health for both men and women, including gender equality. It is, therefore, important to consider evidence that goes beyond modifying behaviour and encompasses the wider social determinants of health. This scoping review includes evidence published in both English and Russian and highlights the similarities and differences found.

1.1.1 Gender and mental health

Gender is well established as a key social determinant of health and well-being, including for men (9). A range of statistics highlights sex differences in mortality, the prevalence of many chronic conditions and mental health problems. For example, women attempt suicide far more frequently than men – yet suicide rates for men are approximately three times those for age-matched women (10), and are even higher in some countries (e.g. 4.5 times higher in the Russian Federation (11)), revealing a gender paradox for suicidal behaviour (12). Similarly, fewer men than women are treated for depression-related disorders (13,14). The overall rates of anxiety and depression are lower in men (15), with 13% of men and 20% of women reporting an episode in the past week in 2007 (16). In the Russian Federation, the risk of developing or triggering depression ranges from 10% to 20% in women and from 5% to 12% in men (17). However, distress may be exhibited more indirectly by men, for example through alcohol and substance misuse and addiction (18,19), anger and aggression towards self and others (20,21) and risk-taking in general (22,23). These differences are influenced by socially constructed gender norms, roles and attributes that intersect with other drivers of inequalities, discrimination and marginalization, such as ethnicity, socioeconomic status, disability, age, geographical location and sexual orientation.

1.1.2 Sociocultural constructions of masculinities

Traditional masculinity norms have been proposed as one reason why so many men are reluctant to report mental health problems or seek professional help (24,25). This is now widely understood in terms of the dominant social norms and cultural stereotypes that, through time, have become associated with men and influence their practices, including health-related practices (22). The term **hegemonic masculinity** is associated with the seminal work of Australian sociologist Raewyn Connell (26,27): it is defined as "the currently most honoured way of being a man" (28) and incorporates the idea that multiple masculinities (and femininities) exist. The work of Connell and other major theorists has been widely translated and has influenced masculinity studies worldwide, including research published in Russian (29–34). However, within the Russian Federation, multidisciplinary analyses informed by intersectional, postcolonial and transnational perspectives in critical studies on men and masculinities compete with other, more psychological, analyses based on sex role theory (35).

Connell has highlighted that power can operate through masculinities: at a given moment in a given context, some men will enact and be privileged by local masculinities, while women and other men will be marginalized (36). Marginalized men include disabled men, who may have little access to valued masculinities, and gay men, who may be subjected to homophobia and judged to fall short of masculine standards. Although the concept of hegemonic masculinity remains popular, including with Russian sociologists (29,37), other theorists emphasize (i) a more positive perspective that highlights how contemporary masculinity can be more caring and inclusive (38,39) or (ii) interactions between traditional and modern ideals of masculinity (40,41). In this context of changing masculinities, it should be acknowledged that some men may in fact prioritize their well-being and adopt healthy masculinities (42,43) or at least adopt some health-promoting behaviours, including exercise, healthy eating and reduced alcohol consumption (9).

The range of masculinities available to men varies between countries and world regions (e.g. within Europe (44)), although there is also evidence of transnational or global masculinities (e.g. among metropolitan business elites (45)). At the same time, it is important to recognize the complexity and plurality of masculinities within countries (e.g. the Russian Federation (46–48)) related to mutually influencing social dimensions (e.g. social class, race, sexual orientation, location (urban vs rural), (un)employment and mobility/migration), the disproportionate impact of important life events on men (e.g. unemployment, injury or incarceration) and the capacity of men to negotiate their own health and well-being, including psychological issues (49–52). Currently in the Russian Federation, men's ideas, practices and models of masculinity are contextualized in relation to post-Soviet political transformations and post-socialist socioeconomic changes (18,38,53), often termed the **men's crisis** (25).

In general, men's mental health suffers in regions with high unemployment and where (i) the sole breadwinner model prevails as a key component of masculinity (e.g. in Spain (54)), (ii) the financial crisis and subsequent austerity measures have had a disproportionate impact on male suicide rates (e.g. in Greece (55)) and (iii) the area in which the men grew up was economically disadvantaged, where men are more prone to substance misuse and psychological difficulties (e.g. in Scotland (United Kingdom) (56)).

1.1.3 Masculinities influence mental health help-seeking

The perception of help-seeking as weakness by some men can cause them to avoid mental health services or can lead to long delays between problem recognition and help-seeking (57,58). Reluctance to seek support can be the result of structural challenges, where help-seeking can quickly lead to labelling and consequent restriction on life choices, making it potentially more difficult to find employment.

It has also been linked to a preference for self-reliance and autonomy among men, features that are traditionally linked to masculinity norms (22). This phenomenon is not confined to western Europe and North America; for example, in the Russian Federation (59):

> [m]en are much less likely to use medical, social and psychological services and generally prefer not to consult doctors and other specialists. As a result, men often experience a delay in diagnosis and do not receive the necessary help in a timely manner. This applies to almost all diseases, as well as to other problems in all categories of men, especially the poor. Studies show that it is difficult for men to ask for help because "they must be strong and proud"; thus, a large gap is formed between men's need for help and men's search for help. This applies not only to medical but also to psychological and social assistance in general.

In men who experience distress, self-medication through excessive alcohol consumption or substance misuse is clearly influenced by traditional masculinity norms (14) but also perhaps by a lack of available, visible, gender-informed therapeutic services to which they can turn in times of need.

However, it would be simplistic to ignore other intersecting factors that affect men's help-seeking for psychological problems. For example, compared with married men, suicidal thoughts and suicide attempts are three times higher in divorced men and two times higher in separated men (where it is linked to consequent social withdrawal and isolation) (60), reinforcing the importance of gender on key life events and transitions. Both suicidal ideation and suicide attempts among men (and women) show a clear inverse correlation with household income: the prevalence of both is lower among those with the highest income and greatest among those with the lowest income (61,62). Thus, economic austerity, unemployment, low-paid unstable work and financial hardship can undermine conventional masculine roles (i.e. as breadwinner or protector), leading to psychological difficulties (63,64). Many countries also report higher suicide rates in male prisoners, who are predominantly young and from disadvantaged backgrounds (65,66). Men also constitute the majority of single homeless people, another group that is vulnerable to mental illness (67).

Variations in mental illness are seen across regions and within groups of men. The prevalence of traditional ideals of masculinity that have become unachievable due to societal changes has clear psychological consequences for men. For example, in the Russian Federation the sole breadwinner model (part of the hegemonic masculine identity) creates in men expectations that, when not fulfilled, provoke frustration and compensatory behaviours that may entail health risk factors (68–70).

> The transformation of Russian society has weakened the social positions of men as breadwinners, providers and protectors. Since conventional gender stereotypes still have a strong influence, the male gender display deteriorates into early male mortality, alcoholism, drug addiction, psychosomatic disorders and increased aggressiveness. But, in general, the problems of men's discrimination are not being brought up for public discussion nor recognized by men themselves.

In regions where gender equality is prioritized, such as the Nordic countries, men find it easier to transition from the sole breadwinner model to a dual earner model, with reported improvements in health and well-being (e.g. in Denmark (71)). Furthermore, in regions where more men progress into higher education, there is a greater tendency for men to seek help for a range of problems (72,73). At community level, there is emerging evidence that interventions to improve men's health and well-being can be effective in engaging men if they involve community members in their design and delivery and are based on locally valued masculinity norms (25,74,75). For example, in many countries, older men who are isolated and vulnerable to mental illness have benefited from the Men's Shed initiative, where the focus is on male camaraderie, making things together (e.g. using carpentry) and supporting each other indirectly – shoulder to shoulder rather than face to face (76).

Intersectional approaches have shown that masculinities intersect with other determinants of difference and inequality related to social class, race, ethnicity, age, sexuality and disability (77,78). Psychological difficulties experienced by minority ethnic men are linked to exposure to racial violence, stigmatization and prejudice (79), while rates of depression, anxiety and attempted suicide are higher in gay men than in heterosexual men (80,81). Recent evidence from non-European settings showed that societal and institutional bias, discrimination and marginalization restricts the access of men and boys to the benefits, opportunities and resources enjoyed by more privileged groups (82,83). The consequent limited range of (toxic) masculine identities might make them less likely to engage with mainstream mental health services, which may be culturally insensitive (20,82,83).

1.1.4 Objectives of this report

No systematic analysis of research in the WHO European Region is yet available on the relationships between sociocultural constructions of masculinities and men's mental health help-seeking behaviour within the wider determinants of health. This report aims to review the best available evidence on how sociocultural constructs of masculinities are associated with men's mental health help-seeking behaviour and proposes a set of policy considerations to support policy-makers in creating programmes geared to enhance the mental health and well-being of men in the Region.

1.2 Methodology

A literature search in March 2019 examined articles published in English or Russian between 1 January 2009 and 1 February 2019 in the peer-reviewed and grey literature. The report was also informed by expert reviewer comments on the first draft and by written and verbal feedback from panel members of the fifth WHO expert group meeting on cultural contexts of health and well-being held in June 2019, which identified further research papers, reports and policy documents for inclusion. The literature search (after removal of duplicates) and additional sources identified 3197 articles in English, of which 155 full-text articles were reviewed, with 23 fulfilling the criteria for inclusion (57,84–105). The literature search (after removal of duplicates) and additional sources identified 399 papers in Russian; of these, 124 underwent a full-text review and 18 articles fulfilled the criteria for inclusion (25,38,49–52,58,75,106–115). A total of 41 papers were included in the scoping review. Further details on the search strategy are provided in Annex 1.

In addition, the identified literature was contextualized based on the authors' knowledge of fields such as the critical study of men and masculinities, gender studies and men's health, paying attention to what was absent or underspecified, and with a focus on culture.

2. RESULTS

Publications in English were from the United States of America ($n = 7$), Canada ($n = 6$), and then Europe ($n = 5$: Sweden, $n = 2$; United Kingdom, $n = 2$; Ireland, $n = 1$) and Australia ($n = 1$); reviews were from the United States ($n = 2$), Canada ($n = 1$) and the United Kingdom ($n = 1$). Publications in Russian were from the Russian Federation ($n = 7$) or specific Russian cities/regions (*oblasts*): St Petersburg ($n = 5$), Kuzbass Region ($n = 2$), Altai Region ($n = 1$), Kaluga ($n = 1$), Ryazan ($n = 1$) and Tomsk ($n = 1$).

Studies published in English reported either qualitative ($n = 8$) or quantitative ($n = 11$) data. Seven qualitative studies used interviews along with a range of analytic techniques, including thematic, phenomenology and discourse analyses; the other reported data from an online forum. In total, the qualitative studies included data from 164 male participants. Of the quantitative studies, seven used masculinity scales and measures of help-seeking; two analysed existing survey datasets; one used an experimental study design; and one used structured interviews and rating scales. The quantitative studies included a total of 10 163 men; most featured men only (two used survey data from men and women). In contrast, most articles in Russian were review-type papers using existing statistical data, with only a few involving data collection. Those using existing data included debates on men's issues and data on men's activism variables ($n = 2$); problem-setting opinion pieces ($n = 2$); quantitative studies based on researcher-generated questionnaires ($n = 4$), thematic analysis ($n = 2$) and review articles ($n = 5$); issue-oriented qualitative studies ($n = 2$); and training manuals related to psychological assistance for male patients, including statements on men's help-seeking behaviour ($n = 1$). Most studies used survey data collected from both men and women.

The review identified intersections between gender and characteristics (e.g. race, sexual orientation and age), life stages and challenges (e.g. young adulthood, middle age and old age) and the wider societal influences on men's health and well-being (e.g. poverty, prejudice and economic insecurity), aligned with the WHO Gender Responsive Assessment Scale (Table 1) **(116)**. Key themes pertaining to the role of masculinities (and wider community-level and societal factors) in inhibiting or facilitating men's help-seeking for mental health problems were highlighted:

- stigma
- tailored support
- community-level interventions

- reframing help-seeking within traditional masculinity norms
- rethinking masculinity, challenging traditional concepts and depictions.

Case studies provide examples of interventions that had improved mental health help-seeking in different groups of men selected from both the English and Russian literature.

Table 1. WHO Gender Responsive Assessment Scale: criteria for assessing programmes and policies

Level	Criteria
1. Gender-unequal	• Perpetuates gender inequality by reinforcing unbalanced norms, roles and relations • Privileges men over women (or vice versa) • Often leads to one sex enjoying more rights or opportunities than the other
2. Gender-blind	• Ignores gender norms, roles and relations • Very often reinforces gender-based discrimination • Ignores differences in opportunities and resource allocation for women and men • Often constructed based on the principle of being "fair" by treating everyone the same
3. Gender-sensitive	• Considers gender norms, roles and relations • Does not address inequality generated by unequal norms, roles or relations • Indicates gender awareness, although often no remedial action is developed
4. Gender-specific	• Considers gender norms, roles and relations for women and men and how they affect access to and control over resources • Considers women's and men's specific needs • Intentionally targets and benefits a specific group of women or men to achieve certain policy or programme goals or meet certain needs • Makes it easier for women and men to fulfil duties that are ascribed to them based on their gender roles

Table 1 contd

5. Gender-transformative	· Considers gender norms, roles and relations for women and men and that these affect access to and control over resources · Considers women's and men's specific needs · Addresses the causes of gender-based health inequities · Includes ways to transform harmful gender norms, roles and relations · Objective is often to promote gender equality · Includes strategies to foster progressive changes in power relationships between women and men

Source: World Health Organization, 2010 (116).

2.1 Stigma around men's mental health issues

2.1.1 Influence of traditional masculinity norms

The evidence overwhelmingly showed that traditional masculinity norms stigmatize help-seeking for mental health problems and limit men's knowledge and capability concerning mental health; these norms vary and operate differently according to individual, interpersonal, community and societal contexts. Although stigma concerning mental health issues is increasingly being debated and challenged in many countries, it remains a powerful deterrent to help-seeking for men (74). In eastern European countries and the Russian Federation, most people have a strong bias against psychologists and psychiatrists, but not towards specialists or any system of detection (117).

Evidence from the Russian Federation described a culture of poor self-care and health literacy in men and a lack of effective training strategies in health care for men (118). The influence of traditional masculinity norms means that many men may experience greater stigma for mental illness (49,50). This is compounded by masculine stereotypes concerning self-reliance, which may deter men from seeking help (50,59,109,112). Norms such as toughness, anti-femininity, emotional control and rationality were seen to inhibit men from disclosing their mental health issues, especially within the wider culture of discomfort and prejudice around such issues (101).

Stigma around mental health may be internalized to produce self-stigma, whereby depressed men consider themselves as not measuring up to masculinity standards and, as a consequence, experience a sense of guilt and failure (85). Evidence from questionnaire-based studies showed that greater adherence to traditional masculinity norms was associated with higher levels of self-stigma (84,86). Evidence from the Russian Federation indicated a clear link between prevailing masculinity ideals and the reluctance/ambivalence of many men to seek help for mental health concerns: men make up only 20% of the client population and drop out of treatment prematurely (Case study 1) (109).

Case study 1. Socially constructed masculinities constrain suicide prevention efforts, Russian Federation

A key study assessed young male respondents' answers to the question "Would you like to consult a psychiatrist, psychotherapist or psychologist" in order to develop a suicidal and psychological profile (110). The researchers also analysed how the parents' contribution to gender socialization shaped the boys' transition into adolescence and young adulthood. They found that some parents undermined their son's mental health by encouraging him to develop an adult degree of self-reliance. In contrast, other parents:

> tried to "tame their child" by all means, that is, to solve all his problems, thereby maintaining the teenager in a more infantile state, which is particularly dangerous where men are considered in terms of their gender identity. The consequent confusion may cause pronounced cognitive dissonance or create a "double clamp" against gender socialization in boys.

> When a man experiences familial prohibition against intimacy (in other words, does not have a trusted person to share his problems with), it becomes very difficult for him to communicate honestly with a specialist who, of course, needs to be trusted. In some cases, a feeling of "Don't do it" might prevent him from taking this essential step. Perhaps the motto of the study group is best phrased as: "It is better to sit, endure and not to stick out".

Boys and young men with familial prohibitions might find help-seeking difficult – and those who do consult professionals might be harshly judged by their peers and family:

> some men are of the opinion that if you are not coping with your difficulties, then you are not a man. And that if you go to a psychologist or psychiatrist, "it means you are a weakling". These thoughts often prevent young men from adequately understanding situations from which they cannot escape on their own.

Case study 1 contd

These prevailing attitudes have consequences for men's mental well-being:

> [they] often experienced feelings of shame, guilt and despair, and persistent remorse. They are also characterized by having a predominance of depressive reactions, feeling that their life lacks meaning, and often experiencing feelings of loneliness.

This case study highlights the importance of early interventions focused on families and the school environment for suicide prevention in boys and young men.

In the Russian Federation, cultural stigma is compounded by limited service provision for mental health problems: general practitioners are not trained to treat problems such as depression, while specialist outpatient services (*dispanseri*) work outside mainstream health-care services and are not equipped to treat large populations (119).

Some reports also identified a specific stigma around medication use for mental health issues: men seemed reluctant to admit to others (especially their male peers) that they were taking tablets (95,96). This was also influenced by masculinity norms such as self-reliance, emotional control, toughness, independence and action orientation. An observational study of reactions to and rankings of mental health labels and sources of support in 85 men in the United States noted that those who adhered to the norm of self-reliance responded more negatively to the prospect of taking medication (97). Evidence from the Russian Federation also revealed notable stigma around visiting mental health services and a preference for seeking advice from friends, if at all, who are ill-equipped to help (110).

2.1.2 Substance abuse and mental health issues

Several quantitative studies confirmed that women are more likely than men to report mental health problems (e.g. in Ireland (87)) and that men who conform more to traditional masculine norms are less likely to seek help (e.g. in the United Kingdom (103) and United States (86)). A questionnaire study of 1051 men and women in the United States found that high scores on toughness were linked to delayed help-seeking for both sexes, but especially for men (89). Evidence also showed that male-specific symptoms of depression-associated aggression, irritability, substance use, risky behaviour and physical complaints, which are not captured by the *Diagnostic and Statistical Manual of Mental Disorders* (120) or existing diagnostic tools (90), can make help-seeking less likely (91). Men in the Russian Federation are more likely to turn to alcohol consumption and drug use than to seek professional help (58). Further, drinking and poor self-care in Russian men have been linked to wider societal factors, including an overemphasis on state-sanctioned health care over individual lifestyle practices, and a smaller middle-class sector compared with western European and North American countries (where middle-class sectors are associated with healthier lifestyles) (121).

Substance abuse is a problem for some marginalized communities of men; for example, in gay, bisexual and transgender men (who disproportionately experience bullying, harassment and hate crimes), self-medication to manage minority stress often exacerbates mental ill health and increases risk of suicide (122). Different groups and subcultures have particular substance use preferences, for example steroid intake in younger men (123) and increased alcohol consumption in older men (124). Other groups vulnerable to substance abuse include homeless men, men in incarceration (106), indigenous men (e.g. native American Indians in the United States) and rural men (82).

The prevalence of substance abuse in marginalized male communities means that the men themselves, their friends and family, and even health professionals may not interpret this as a sign of mental health problems. This problem may be compounded by limited access to visible, culturally acceptable therapeutic services, leading to delays in help-seeking for these men: the increased risk of depression combined with a more negative attitude toward help-seeking has been described as double jeopardy (101,125). Such men may only decide to seek help following a crisis (e.g. a relationship breakdown) or after experiencing physical symptoms attributable to mental health issues (e.g. panic attacks (92)).

2.1.3 Stigma in male-dominated environments

In particular contexts, local gendered ideals and practices make it especially difficult for men to signal mental health issues. For example, a theoretical analysis suggested that military cultures discourage emotional disclosure through a combination of hypermasculine and working-class norms that promote stoicism, actions over words, denial of pain or weakness, and physical robustness (93). Russian analyses made similar findings concerning military veterans (126), and post-traumatic stress disorder exposure is now acknowledged to be linked to military combat (127) as well as to other traumas such as childhood sexual abuse and experiences of interpersonal violence. It is also increasingly recognized that historical and race-based mistreatment and victimization can have similar consequences for ethnic minority and indigenous men (128).

Men working in other traditionally male-dominated fields (e.g. the fire brigade (129)) may also encounter masculine norms that inhibit displays of vulnerability. Moreover, men may feel pressure to prioritize work commitments over family time and personal well-being, especially in male-dominated industries such as construction (130). Similarly, sporting cultures can inhibit emotional disclosure and help-seeking through promoting mental toughness, competitiveness, playing through pain, and controlled aggression. In a qualitative interview study of eight elite varsity football players in Canada (mean age, 22 years), participants' reluctance to disclose their mental health issues was linked to protecting their status, popularity and performance within the team, with those reporting such issues being viewed as weak, fearful of competition and compromising the team spirit and success (94).

Evidence also indicated that boys and men are particularly concerned that their male peers may react unfavourably to a disclosure of psychological distress (i.e. think less of them or judge them critically) (92,95). Thus, stigma around mental illness might be reinforced and policed by other men (or at least by the perception that other men would respond negatively), which discourages men from disclosing their psychological difficulties, at least in all-male group situations such as bars (92).

2.1.4 Stigmatizing environments for boys

Institutional contexts in which traditional masculinity norms operate to police male identities and practices include mixed-sex environments. For example, in school settings the dominant heteromasculine standards prescribe a restricted range of damaging (or toxic) behaviours, including homophobic and sexist behaviour (131). A recent European Union-funded study of young people in five European countries (Bulgaria, England (United Kingdom), Italy, Latvia and Slovenia) highlighted pervasive sexual bullying whereby boys perceived to deviate from heteromasculine standards were subjected to ridicule and sanctions (131), whereas girls were routinely sexually objectified and pressurized for sex (e.g. in Spain (131,132), the United Kingdom (133) and the United States (134)). Thus, being a victim of bullying is strongly linked to mental health problems, for example in young people who are lesbian, gay, bisexual, transgender or queer; however, young people who bully others are also at risk of mental illness, since violence against others tends to stem from personal experiences of aggression, social exclusion and disadvantage (80,135,136). Such evidence points to the potential of school- and youth centre-based interventions to promote tolerance, inclusivity and positive gender identities. The recent WHO strategy and report on men's health in the WHO European Region identified education on health, well-being and gender equality as a priority for boys and young men (3,5).

Within the family, parenting of boys may reproduce and reinforce restrictive masculinities. Several Russian reports considered gender role socialization for boys as key to understanding how their sociocultural environment influences the appropriation of men's attitudes towards help-seeking behaviours. Child-rearing practices and family traditions were found to influence boys, adolescents and men's attitudes and behaviours towards mental health help-seeking. For example, cultural stereotypes promoted by boys' parents propagated the myth of the "real man" (111). Approaches to analysing and revising this myth include counselling sessions informed by a narrative approach (111,137,138).

2.1.5 Marginalized and vulnerable groups

Help-seeking was found to be more challenging for men in specific disadvantaged groups. A meta-ethnography review of 51 qualitative studies highlighted intersections between gender, ethnicity and sexuality, and reported that help-seeking was lower in men in minority groups, including refugee and migrant, minority ethnic, indigenous, gay, bisexual and rural men (98). In general, difficulties in help-seeking were linked to cultural norms (e.g. family-based shame associated with mental illness), social exclusion and experiences of prejudice and discrimination (e.g. racism or homophobia). A qualitative interview study of 32 Canadian farmers reported that barriers to help-seeking included pride and ignorance about mental health and the available support (99). This was confirmed by survey data: quantitative data from 4825 men suggested that African-American and Mexican-American men are less likely to seek help and have less access to culturally competent health-care providers, and that men from lower lower-socioeconomic status backgrounds are also less likely to seek help (87,100,101).

A previous Health Evidence Network report described the barriers to accessing mental health care encountered by migrants in the WHO European Region (139). Evidence from the Russian Federation similarly showed that social exclusion of refugee and migrant men (who are mainly from central Asian countries (140)) helps to explain their lack of engagement with therapeutic services (141): they do not trust government and public organizations but instead regard their friends, relatives or partners within migration networks as valid sources of support and advice. Conversely, for some ethnic minority groups, migration may have a disruptive impact on their community values, traditions and well-being. For indigenous men of the Tomsk and Tyumen *oblasts* and Altai Region, Buryatia Republic, Chukotka Autonomous Region, Tuva Republic and Sakha Republic, the most significant causes of mental health imbalance were reported as separation from the family environment, loss of sociocultural traditions and the destabilizing influence of refugees and migrants. The most vulnerable group was men under 40 years of age who were living in a mixed family, not working in traditional types of employment and with social benefits as the main sources of income; men in this group were at risk of alcoholism and behavioural disorders (142). In addition, men returning from combat zones face multiple challenges in adjusting to their social environment, accessing employment opportunities and facing threats to their well-being. For example, in the former Yugoslav states that were undergoing post-socialist economic and societal transformations, former soldiers faced unemployment and were consequently unable to perform the traditional roles of breadwinner and protector, which were increasingly valued as nationalistic identities become more firmly established (143,144). Outside this context, a number of other nations are also currently witnessing discourses around men in crisis, anti-feminist rhetoric and precarious masculinity (145,146).

2.1.6 Poor health literacy

Constraints against help-seeking are also linked to limited mental health literacy: men may have a poor understanding of mental health; lack the vocabulary or confidence to articulate emotional distress; misinterpret or minimize psychological symptoms; and lack knowledge about the available sources of support (92,95,98,99,101–103). For example, an analysis of Canadian survey data featuring responses from 452 men found that over 40% felt that they were not well informed about mental illness (102). An interview study of Australian men reported a simplistic, distorted understanding of mental illness, featuring hallucinations, hearing voices and extreme behaviour (92). In a Swedish interview study of 13 young urban men, participants agreed that men are not socialized to understand, notice or articulate difficult emotions (95).

This lack of knowledge is clearly linked to traditional masculinity norms, particularly emotional control, strength, rationality and independence. Poor mental health literacy in men may be informed by familial, occupational, cultural and regional norms that discourage discourse about psychological issues, for example in male-dominated workplaces (e.g. construction sites (130)) and in working-class communities, where men may prioritize humour, breadwinning and protecting others (147). More broadly, the resources and cultural capital required to access information, advice and support on mental health issues may not be available to men in disadvantaged communities, while health services may not openly offer or promote culturally acceptable interventions.

2.2 Support tailored to the needs of diverse groups of men

Despite the strong link between traditional masculinity norms and poor mental health literacy and a reluctance to seek help, some evidence indicated that masculinity-framed interventions can encourage men to access and engage with therapeutic services. Interventions were most effective when their content and presentation were targeted to a specific group of men; for example, the needs of sexual minority men may differ from those of heterosexual men (82). Therefore, to be most effective, interventions should include factors other than gender (masculinity) and ideally be designed through consultation with relevant community groups and members (74,109). This section describes how masculinities contribute to successful approaches to men's mental health promotion; the intersections between gender and other identity dimensions; and how local cultural norms, inequalities and social exclusion are being addressed.

2.2.1 Support from significant others

In general, men are more willing to disclose their emotional issues in communities where help-seeking is normative and appropriate support is readily available. Help-seeking by men may be facilitated by supportive environments in which emotional communication is normalized and validated (25,85). More specific evidence indicates that men can be persuaded to seek help by significant others (wives/partners, parents) and within trusted communities (groups/peers within the local neighbourhood; fellow members of social/sport clubs). Several papers cited the important role of female partners in encouraging men to disclose their psychological problems and prompting them to seek help. A questionnaire study of 136 rodeo cowboys in the United States reported a preference for talking things over with female partners over all other options (i.e. talking to an expert, joining an Internet forum or attending a relevant class/workshop) (91). An analysis of pre-existing data from the National Psychological Well-being and Distress Survey in Ireland found that male respondents currently in relationships with women were three times more likely to seek help compared with men living by themselves (87). A qualitative interview study of Australian men described the key involvement of wives and girlfriends in prompting help-seeking – with men noting that they might have done nothing without such support (92). This denotes a guarded vulnerability in which men only reveal their problems to select, trusted others so as to preserve their masculine identity (57). However, contradictory evidence was also found: an interview study of American men reported that respondents reacted more positively to the suggestion to seek professional treatment when made by a psychotherapist than by a medical doctor or romantic partner (97).

For younger men, mothers may be key figures in prompting help-seeking and may even physically escort them to the health centre: in the case of one young Swedish man, his mother called the service provider and took him there (95). Fathers were notably absent from these scenarios; however, as new generations of men transition to more-involved models of fatherhood, boys and young men might feel equally at ease disclosing their mental health problems to fathers as to mothers. Engaging fathers in this form of emotional labour would require supportive government policies concerning parental leave, free childcare, flexible working patterns and gender equality more generally (5).

2.2.2 Online support

Growing evidence indicates that many men are engaging with online resources to find out more about mental health issues, including advice on mitigating their problems. A small Swedish study highlighted the use of the Internet by six male interviewees aged in their 20s in a self-management approach to seek information and advice and, where suitable, incorporate this into their lifestyle practices, in alignment with traditional masculinity norms around self-reliance, autonomy and rationality (104). Other men may actually disclose their issues online and seek help anonymously, for example within relevant forums where they can elicit peer support without the risk of losing face or having their masculinity questioned (92,105). In an interview study, a group of Australian men reported that finding out about peers with similar problems online proved helpful by reminding them they are not alone (92). An analysis of online forum interactions involving British men experiencing depression found that the men were concerned to present themselves as having gone to great lengths to manage their problems themselves before seeking help, highlighting the continued influence of traditional masculinity norms such as self-reliance (105).

A clear benefit of anonymous support is that men feel able to maintain control over their situation (85). Nowadays, many such forums and websites hosted in different countries focus on diverse mental health issues and distinct groups of men: some provide support to men experiencing depression and suicidality (e.g. Campaign Against Living Miserably (CALM): Case study 2) while others focus on other problems. For example, men with eating disorders must cope with its dominant cultural and media representations as a women's illness (150). An online community in the United Kingdom dedicated to supporting men with experience of eating disorders offers help and support and features testimonies from men telling their stories (151). Other online sites focus on supporting men struggling with a range of medical issues that affect their well-being, including different forms of cancer (152), infertility (153) and obesity (154). Such websites seem to attract a lot of traffic and engagement, but as yet evidence of impact is sparse.

> Case study 2. CALM offers online support to suicidal and distressed men, United Kingdom
>
> CALM is a suicide prevention organization that initially targeted young men but recently expanded its remit to include all men (148). There is a focus on using everyday, nonmedical language (e.g. "feeling shit" rather than "being depressed") to connect with men. Consistent with evidence that role models who exhibit masculinity capital can influence men's help-seeking behaviour (149), CALM recruits high-profile musicians, actors and comedians as ambassadors to communicate with men using straightforward terms rather than psychological language. Moreover, recognizing that men can struggle to talk openly about mental health issues with friends and family and to seek help, CALM offers free, confidential and anonymous helpline and webchat services, which enables men to retain a sense of personal control. The organization promotes men's mental health in community venues ranging from prisons to universities and workplaces, where it signposts relevant services. It also carries out campaigning activities that challenge traditional notions of masculinity and encourage help-seeking with the help of ambassadors:
>
>> We campaign with media partners, brands and ambassadors to spread awareness of suicide and its devastating impact with campaigns like #Project84, #DontBottleItUp and The Best Man Project. We challenge boring male stereotypes and encourage positive behavioural change and help-seeking behaviour, using cultural touch points like art, music, sport and comedy.

2.2 3 Role models

Other evidence indicates that men can be encouraged to seek help for their mental health issues through endorsement of help-seeking by familiar role models, including members of their community or respected male public figures. However, to be effective, the role models must be perceived as credible through having accrued sufficient masculinity capital (so-called man points), that is, men perceived to embody valued masculine attributes (149). For example, an interview study of

21 college men experiencing depression reported the potential value of other (masculine) men expressing psychological difficulties and promoting help-seeking (96). A man who is perceived to be traditionally masculine (e.g. in terms of his physical stature) and is prepared to display vulnerability and promote help-seeking for emotional problems may be able to influence other men to do so. Other role models may be respected because of their work achievements. For example, an interview study of 32 farmers reported the positive reception of a news story featuring a successful farmer disclosing his mental health difficulties, with interviewees expressing sympathy and support (99).

Clearly, different role models will resonate with different groups of men with shared identity, occupation or leisure interests. The world of sport increasingly provides role models for many men. For example, Australian interviewees made positive references to displays of vulnerability by various high-profile sportsmen (92). Similarly, a Canadian study of varsity footballers highlighted the importance of masculinity capital (i.e. being able to command respect from one's peers) when sportsmen talk about their emotional problems (94). The evidence suggests that men who command respect from other men, whether through success in valued masculine domains (e.g. work or sport) or simple masculine embodiment, can play a key role in reaching men and encouraging help-seeking for psychological problems. Importantly, more diverse role models are needed for disadvantaged and minority men. Currently, elite sport does not provide many role models for gay, bisexual and transgender men. For example, despite recent initiatives to tackle homophobia, no top-level soccer player is currently out in the United Kingdom, and prejudice against sexual minority men continues within elite and amateur sport internationally (155).

2.3 Community-level interventions

2.3.1 Interventions for hard-to-reach groups

Efforts have recently been made to develop community-based initiatives targeting hard-to-reach men in different regions. For example, older men living alone following marital breakdown or bereavement (or even through choice) may be at risk of declining mental health and social isolation and, therefore, in need of special consideration for interventions. One success story is the Men's Sheds movement (Case study 3), which focuses on older, isolated men at risk of mental illness, often in economically deprived and/or geographically remote neighbourhoods (156). Here, community venues are used as spaces for men to congregate and work together on projects, while building social connections and improving well-being in the process.

Community-based initiatives also include crisis centres for men in the Russian Federation (Case study 4). Other community-based initiatives may use sport to attract men: even when an initiative focuses on physical health, there is evidence of mental health gains (160). Interventions are generally tailored to particular groups. For example, programmes for military veterans, a predominantly male population, work well when fellow veterans are involved in the design and management and when insider language, customs and humour are accommodated (161). Emerging initiatives focused on diverse minority communities are tackling cultural issues pertaining to health and well-being. In the United Kingdom, a number of recent newspaper articles, funded projects and community programmes have focused on Muslim men, mixed race men and Afro-Caribbean men (Case study 5).

> Case study 3. Men's Sheds bring older, isolated men together, United Kingdom
>
> Men's Sheds Associations work in many countries to engage older, isolated men and connect them with their peers in order to improve their well-being (156). Broadly, they are a form of community-based mental health provision (although not presented as such) that taps into masculinity norms concerning pragmatism, work, homosociality (i.e. social interactions between men) and banter. Such initiatives characterize a shoulder-to-shoulder rather than face-to-face approach, where men share their emotions indirectly in the context of performing an activity (76). The website states:
>
>> For a long time, research has shown the negative impact of loneliness and isolation on a person's health and well-being. Recently we have seen more evidence come to light that shows loneliness and isolation can be as hazardous to our health as obesity and excessive smoking. Surveys from mental health charities are finding that millions of people report feeling lonely on a daily basis. Men's Sheds are vital.
>
> Men typically find it more difficult than women to build social connections and, unlike women of a similar age, fewer older men have networks of friends and rarely share personal concerns about health and other personal worries (74). For some men, but not all, retirement can feel like a loss of personal identity and purpose. Men's Sheds can provide a place to meet like-minded people and have someone to share your worries with; have fun, share skills and knowledge; and gain a renewed sense of purpose and of belonging. As a by-product, they reduce isolation and feelings of loneliness, allow men to deal more easily with mental health challenges and remain independent; rebuild communities; and, in many cases, they save men's lives.

Case study 4. Men's crisis centres help the most vulnerable men, Russian Federation

In the Russian Federation, various crisis centres offer men psychological support alongside medical and legal assistance. For example, the Altai Regional Crisis Centre for Men explicitly sets out to challenge certain traditional masculinity ideals (157):

> The purpose: to support the physical, mental and social health of men of working age through the provision of social, psychological, sociomedical, legal assistance to men in crisis …
>
> It is generally believed that strong men do not need support because they are naturally endowed with the ability to stoically face all difficulties and cope with emerging problems. This myth does not help a man at all. On the contrary, it can aggravate his emotional state if he cannot immediately resolve the difficult situation he finds himself in. Psychological counselling … creates the conditions for acquiring new knowledge and skills to address men's existing problems.
>
> The aim of the Centre is to preserve, maintain and restore the mental and social health of boys and men living in the Altai Region.

Other centres provide support for specific populations of men, for example victims of physical, sexual or psychological violence; the "Colon" Crisis Centre for Male Victims of Violence in St Petersburg (158) states, "Every day we help men from different cities to obtain free, anonymous psychological and legal help in our centre".

The Crisis Centre for Men in Syktyvkar (State Budgetary Institution of the Komi Republic "Centre for the social rehabilitation of homeless, unemployed persons in Syktyvkar"), which supports men in desperate circumstances (159), works to:

> solve problems and provide social protection for men trapped in difficult life situations: homeless men, ex-prisoners and war veterans. The range of social services includes legal, psychological and medical help.

As this type of centre caters for a range of issues, the reason for men's attendance will not be obvious to others, resulting in less stigma.

Case study 5. Culture, religion and ethnic minorities: mental health promotion for men from south Asian backgrounds, United Kingdom

In the United Kingdom, more academic attention has recently focused on the role of culture in shaping ethnic minority men's (poor) help-seeking and mental health (135). There has also been some media coverage of cultural issues and mental health. For example, in a newspaper article in 2019, a prominent Muslim general practitioner, Mohammedabbas Khaki, reflected on the influence of culture and religion on Muslim men's mental health practices (162):

> We've inherited sometimes noble, often harmful ideals of traditional masculinity, of the importance of stoicism, of being seen as the unbreakable, impenetrable provider without weakness. Other downright dangerous traditional views also persist. Blame is often placed on the person who is depressed, and their faith questioned as if it is an issue of belief. Mental illness is often seen as a weakness. Often, community members believe that because depression isn't visible, it is simply not real. In fact it speaks volumes that the word "depression" doesn't even exist in many of the South Asian languages most widely spoken by British Muslims. ... To Muslim communities and community leaders, it is time that we addressed the issues that exist head on, to address taboos and to support the congregation with their health needs. Moreover, there should be culturally competent mental health provision that caters to BAME [Black, Asian and minority ethnic] experiences. These services should provide holistic health and wellbeing support from the community, for the community.

A recent initiative specifically focused on the mental health of British Punjabi men (second-generation migrants from the Punjab region in north-western India and eastern Pakistan, where the main religion is Sikhism) (163). Recognizing the culturally enforced silence concerning male mental health, the initiative encourages men to share their mental health stories and opinions online in the hope that more Punjabi men will seek help and engage with mental health services. One participant wrote that:

> [m]ental health issues in the Punjabi community are often only treated in social contexts; the individual is forgotten, as he will only bring shame upon the family. There are also other social interpretations of mental

Case study 5 contd

> health, which are just as damaging to the Punjabi and Sikh diaspora: mental health issues are effeminate – not remotely masculine and strong. Mental health issues are "white people's problems" – Indians just deal with their issues quietly. Mental health issues are religiously prohibited – Sikhs are supposed to be in good spirits. Since these are social interpretations, however, it is possible to offer re-interpretations of these problems, eliminating social and cultural stigma, so the individual becomes visible.

2.3.2 Interventions for boys and young men

A WHO priority for men's health and well-being in the European Region relates to early interventions for boys and young men around mental health, gender equality and positive masculinities (5). Despite a growing literature on boyhood studies and young masculinities, there has as yet been little focus on mental health. There is, therefore, potential to develop interventions involving young people (e.g. in school and youth centre settings) and to include well-being as a cornerstone of personal, social and health education. In the United Kingdom and elsewhere, various local and regional initiatives focus on specific issues, including body image, bullying and equality, to promote the mental health of young people; indeed, some schools now provide sessions on mindfulness, yoga and the natural environment to encourage healthy minds (e.g. PSHE Association (164)). For some boys and young men, education and well-being may be compromised by online activities, including gaming, social media and consumption of pornography (165) – all of which need to be addressed within schools and youth centres. Some programmes also explicitly tackle gender identity, relations and equality. For example, the Good Lad Initiative in the United Kingdom is a nongovernmental organization that conducts workshops with male pupils designed to debate and question restrictive (i.e. toxic) masculinities and promote more positive, inclusive and caring masculinities (166). In addition, some bullying prevention programmes incorporate gender as a key focus; for example, in an European Union-funded project on young people and sexual bullying (131), the research team developed a series of exercises with young people that encouraged critical thinking and behaviour change concerning homophobic and sexist practices (167). WHO has also stressed the importance of gender, sex and relationship education and of equipping young people with the skills to make positive choices (168).

Interesting anti-bullying methods are used in Kazakhstan, which has no special anti-bullying rules in schools. Cases of bullying are considered by the Council of Fathers at the request of a teacher or pupil-victim to ensure that the bully is stopped and punished (169). Local government leaders are also involved in such issues. The Russian Federation also has a number of local and regional anti-bullying programmes and initiatives. As part of a federal programme of mental health services, a national Federal Resource Centre (to be completed by 2025) is planned for teachers and psychologists working in the education system. The Centre will organize a programme to prevent bullying, aggressive and suicidal behaviour for children in schools (170).

Young people who do well educationally are more likely to enjoy better health and well-being (171,172). However, boys and young men are known to perform worse at school than their female counterparts (173), are more likely to leave education early and less likely to engage in further training or gain employment (i.e. to be NEET (young people not in education, employment or training)) (174). This is more likely to be the case for young men and women from marginalized groups (e.g. Roma), with disabilities and from ethnic minorities (175), who may experience institutional bias, microaggression and a lack of cultural recognition within the school environment (82). Consequently, these young men are at risk of coming into contact with the criminal justice system, experiencing violence and substance abuse, and suffering poor mental health (135).

2.3.3 Interventions for fathers

Fatherhood provides another opportunity for intervention. Increasing evidence shows that more-involved fathers enjoy better mental health, and that these benefits are transferred to their partners and children (176). In addition, boys with caring fathers are more likely to become caring fathers themselves (72). Obviously, cultural norms and expectations influence the degree of paternal involvement (108,111), but other institutional and societal factors are also important, including workplace policies on parental leave and flexible working, the availability of free childcare, and wider gender equality and family policies (176). The Russian Federation has been experiencing a trend towards more-involved fathers that is associated with a transformation in masculinity norms (177).

The modern phenomenon of the more-involved father has also been noted in refugee and migrant communities and can be linked to cultural integration (e.g. in Polish migrants (178)). Labour migration in the European Union has been linked to the reaffirmation of traditional masculinity ideals in both host and recipient cultures (179). Interestingly, some religions (e.g. the Russian Orthodox Church) have been intensively rejuvenated through promoting traditional values within which a model of responsible masculinity and fatherhood is promoted as "conservative norm protagonism" (180).

2.3.4 Interventions for marginalized groups

Confidential services are also needed for men in desperation who have not had the good fortune to benefit from peer, familial, institutional or community assistance. Such groups of marginalized men include ex-offenders struggling to adapt to life outside prison, homeless men, male victims of violence and abuse, and men addicted to alcohol or other substances (75,109). In Russian-speaking countries, where mental illness and men's disclosure of emotional problems is stigmatized, crisis centres established to help men in extreme difficulty offer advice to practitioners working with men based on evidence from the Russian Federation and beyond (75,109).

2.4 Reframing help-seeking within traditional masculinity norms

Help-seeking is not a one-time, personal decision; rather, it is best conceived as a dynamic interaction between individuals, significant others and available mental health services situated within wider societal parameters (e.g. national health budgets, social exclusion levels or employment levels) (181). Although traditional masculinity norms (e.g. self-reliance, difficulty in expressing emotions, and autonomy) can constrain men's help-seeking for psychological problems, recent research efforts have focused on developing and evaluating male-friendly interventions to improve help-seeking by leveraging these masculinity norms.

2.4.1 Gender-sensitive language in mental health promotion

A study of 1397 men with depression who had not sought help for their condition found that a male-sensitive brochure was more effective than previous brochures in changing their attitudes towards seeking counselling (84). Informed by theory and research on masculinity and mental health, the brochure featured nonmedical, pragmatic language; an emphasis on problem-solving; and testimonials with images of stereotypical men. This research highlights the importance of language in engaging men by replacing medicalized or psychological terminology (which men may consider effeminate) with less pathologizing and more familiar, acceptable language (e.g. stressed, burnt out or overwhelmed) (98,104). Through careful attention to language within mental health promotion materials, men's limited mental health literacy might be addressed in an appropriate, comfortable and safe way. The language and presentation should be tailored to specific groups of men. For example, staff/interpreters who speak the relevant language and promotion materials in different languages are essential to engage refugee and migrant men in mental health services. The customs, traditions and values of particular ethnic communities should also be acknowledged, for example their religious/spiritual beliefs, traditional familial roles and responsibilities, and main challenges and resources (see Case study 5). For younger men in general, social media has been suggested as a fruitful avenue for mental health promotion. There have been some general initiatives in this area but there is a need for specific interventions that work for specific groups, such as young gay men, young Asian men or young disabled men, and for subgroups such as young gay Asian men.

2.4.2 Gender-specific symptoms can mask mental health issues

Several papers highlighted that men with mental health conditions may experience non-traditional symptoms that are not routinely recognized in diagnosis. For example, symptoms such as aggression, irritability, substance use, risk-taking and somatic complaints might reduce help-seeking in men with depression (91). To address this problem, efforts have been made to construct diagnostic tools to more efficiently identify (male) depression (114,182).

2.4.3 Redesigning traditional masculinity ideals in mental health interventions

Successful initiatives can reframe traditional concepts of masculinity by presenting help-seeking as a masculine norm rather than a feminine stereotype. For example, the brochure study (section 2.4.1) reframed help-seeking so that, instead of being associated with fragility, femininity or failure, it was more constructively presented as the more responsible, rational, brave and independent option – thereby maintaining traditional masculinity ideals (84). Reframing has also been reported in men who have engaged with services. For example, in an interview study of depressed men in Canada, some participants reformulated help-seeking as an active, rational, decisive move (57).

Mental health services can try to engage men by deploying traditional masculinity ideals. For example, men may respond more positively when services involve strength-based action rather than "just talking" (which men may associate with femininity and passivity) (101). One study reported a marked preference in men for cognitive behavioural therapy, with an emphasis on action (57); an interviewee in another study viewed therapy as a means of regaining autonomy (85). Therefore, although engagement with services may be construed as potentially emasculating, the process can be reconstructed in traditionally masculine terms (e.g. action-focused) and/or as a route to regaining valued masculine attributes (e.g. independence). More generally, men may need to negotiate the transition from self-management to engagement with health-care services (95). Conversely, linking common mental health problems with factors beyond the individual's control, whether biological (genetics, neurochemistry), experiential (trauma, isolation) or societal (availability of services, social exclusion), may reassure some men and encourage their engagement (84), although resistance to medication may persist (95). A model emphasizing masculinity-related virtues may be more effective in engaging men who respond to factors influencing traditional masculinities. Consequently, a therapeutic approach featuring collaboration, pragmatic focus and goal-setting may well work for some men – ultimately, men will seek help if it is accessible, appropriate and engaging (101). Interventions should also be informed by the target community of men; for example, what works for traumatized military veterans may not work so well for young men with body image issues.

2.5 Rethinking masculinity?

2.5.1 Challenging traditional concepts of masculinity

High conformity to masculine norms is known to correlate with reduced help-seeking (97). It, therefore, follows that men who do not identify strongly with traditional masculinity are more likely to seek help. The analysis showed that some groups of men are more likely to question, rework or reject conventional notions of masculinity, including those from more socially privileged groups, who have greater resources and (masculinity) capital (87), and those who have experience or knowledge of mental health issues, either personally or within their family or social network (38,96).

In one study, a middle-class interviewee predicted that disclosure of his mental health issues would be received differently by his "white-collar" versus "blue-collar" peers, and that he would receive more understanding and sympathy from the former (85). In an interview study of depressed college men, one participant acknowledged that his openness to emotional expression was not normative but was borne from family experience (96). In another interview study, some men said they were open to talking things through with a health professional and appreciated being listened to and cared for, which represents a traditionally more feminine position (57). In an interview study, young urban Swedish men with depression described their experience of coping with mental illness as occurring alongside a process of redefining masculine identity to accommodate emotional well-being, including being entitled to feel vulnerable (95). Russian analyses also reported that men's experiences of mental illness may prompt a reconsideration of masculine stereotypes (38) and a more positive attitude towards help-seeking (11).

2.5.2 Changing depictions of masculinity in popular culture

Popular culture has an important role in propagating particular masculinities in different geographical regions. Although every region features a complex array of gendered signifiers, some interesting patterns and developments were noted. Evidence from the Russian Federation showed that popular male icons include stars of western European and North American action movies, who exhibit hegemonic masculinity through behaviours such as explicitly reserved brutality, courage, risk-taking, resilience, active sexuality and an individual code of honour (e.g. Jason Statham). Importantly, physical health, elegance and commitment to exclusively male friendship form part of his masculinity norm package. In contrast, the Russian national film industry more actively promotes the paternalist image of male brotherhood (i.e. commitment to male power, rationality, risk-taking and solidarity for the sake of a just cause) (183,184). At the same time, contemporary models of masculinity that include the values of taking part in sport, physical health care, involved fatherhood, pro-family values and traditional collective male hobbies (fishing and hunting) are also popular.

In some countries such as the United States, a widespread cultural debate about changing masculinities is taking place in the wake of high-profile social media campaigns such as #metoo. Although this has led to a backlash from various men's rights organizations and the populist media, the movement towards more positive, progressive masculinities is evident (185). More mature, nuanced depictions of masculinities are also becoming more evident in popular culture, including in best-selling books (e.g. *How Not to be a Boy* (186)) and documentaries (e.g. *All Man: Grayson Perry on Masculinity* (187)). Interestingly, some manufacturers of male grooming products are retreating from macho advertising towards depicting more inclusive forms of masculinity (Case study 6). In the Russian Federation, morning prime time on the national television channels, Channel 1 Russia and VGTRK (All-Russia State Television and Radio Broadcasting Company), is given to the health literacy and health promotion programmes (e.g. *Health, It's Great to Live!*, and *About the Most Important Things*), which regularly cover the questions and issues related to masculinity and aspects of men's health and well-being.

Contemporary Russian films have also addressed the theme of masculinity crisis, with reference to either ethnicity (Solbon Lygdenov's 2013 film, *Bulag – the Sacred Spring*, about the rural Buryat community (190)) or men in a class struggle (Yurii Bykov's 2018 film, *The Factory* (191)).

Case study 6. Changing representations of masculinity within the male grooming industry

A recent high-profile advertising campaign by the global shaving brand Gillette presented a short film critiquing toxic masculinity (i.e. male violence, sexual harassment) and promoting instead a new, more caring form of masculinity. In the process, the brand's original slogan "The Best a Man Can Get" was replaced by "The Best a Man Can Be". A companion website explained the thinking behind the campaign (188):

> It's time we acknowledge that brands, like ours, play a role in influencing culture. And as a company that encourages men to be their best, we have a responsibility to make sure we are promoting positive, attainable, inclusive and healthy versions of what it means to be a man. With that in mind, we have spent the last few months taking a hard look at our past and coming communication and reflecting on the types of men and behaviours we want to celebrate. We're inviting all men along this journey with us – to strive to be better, to make us better, and to help each other be better.
>
> From today on, we pledge to actively challenge the stereotypes and expectations of what it means to be a man everywhere you see Gillette.

The campaign has generated a lot of debate within mainstream and social media, receiving much praise but also accusations of undermining men and masculinity. Despite accusations of virtue signalling (i.e. supporting a particular position for social approval rather than genuine belief), the company has pledged to donate US$ 1 million per year to non-profit-making organizations working with boys and young men to promote positive masculinities. Follow-up promotions have striven to demonstrate diverse masculinities, including a Facebook video featuring a transgender man learning to shave from his father.

Case study 6 contd

Other male grooming companies are also engaged in presenting new images and stories concerning contemporary masculinity and well-being, including the Lynx (also known as Axe) "Men in Progress" video project (189):

> We know that young men can find it hard to express themselves. We want to help guys talk about the things that matter to them, from feelings, emotions and relationships, to the things that drive them. So we've created "Men in Progress", a series of videos where we talk to a group of very different guys and explore what masculinity means to them.

Such high-profile campaigns contribute to debates about modern masculinities and mental health by providing resources, role models and images that may particularly appeal to boys and young men.

3. DISCUSSION

3.1 Strengths and limitations of this review

A strength of the review is its focus on evidence published both in English and in Russian because literature on masculinities and men's well-being in the Russian Federation is not widely known. Only articles published between January 2009 and February 2019 were included in order to prioritize contemporary research: papers published before 2009 almost exclusively focus on traditional masculinity as undermining mental health, whereas those published since 2009 provide more sophisticated analyses that include the positive impacts of masculinity. However, few studies identified in Russian focused on men's help-seeking behaviour in terms of mental health or featured original data collection and analysis. Although there were no geographical limitations, all articles in Russian were from the Russian Federation, and articles in English were highly skewed towards North America (Canada and the United States) and Australia, where research into men's health is well established. Most European articles were from the United Kingdom, despite searching for reports from other European countries. Therefore, future work could include searches for relevant articles published in languages other than English and Russian.

The review also included a range of different methodologies (qualitative, quantitative, mixed methods), as well as some review papers and commentaries. However, as a scoping review, it did not involve a rigorous assessment of the quality of the articles included, and a more systematic review may have excluded some articles and identified further relevant articles for inclusion. Nevertheless, all studies included in the review contributed to addressing the synthesis question, regardless of their sample size or scope, and key recurring themes were identified across the literature.

Much of the literature used questionnaires and constructs designed by psychologists. This was perhaps inevitable given the tight focus of the synthesis question, but a future review could also consider evidence produced by researchers working on masculinity within the fields of gender studies, sociology and public health. However, review of the first draft of the report by independent experts meant that the initial scope was broadened to incorporate socioeconomic, cultural and environmental constraints for men's help-seeking.

3.2 Beyond masculinities: a need for further research

3.2.1 Barriers to men's mental health help-seeking

Overall, the review found that traditional masculinity norms, cultural stereotypes and gender roles inhibit men from seeking help for psychological problems, although effective facilitators to increase mental health help-seeking in men were also identified. Men are overrepresented in some extremely vulnerable populations, such as prisoner and homeless communities. Publications in English provided clear evidence that experiences of violence, abuse and prejudice affect the life chances and mental health of sexual and ethnic minority men (82); in contrast, the Russian literature included only a few, rather general, studies of sexual minority men's mental health and well-being (192). Other vulnerable groups of men were identified as indigenous, refugee and migrant, rural and disabled men (5). Men with multiple disadvantages may be especially at risk (i.e. members of multiple groups such as gay, black, indigenous and/or rural men). The impact of traditional masculinity norms on particular life events and transitions (e.g. bullying; leaving home; being unemployed or in precarious, low-paid work; becoming a father; falling ill; separation/divorce or bereavement; and retirement) can make boys and men vulnerable to social isolation, substance misuse and psychological difficulties (83,114). However, the review found that community, cultural, economic and structural forces are also at play, including the availability of effective services to help deal with poverty, social exclusion and stigma. Therefore, new gender-transformative interventions (116) should consider the link between gender and the wider life contexts of diverse groups of men (and women).

Some countries have initiated a national men's health policy to help to address the multiple factors that affect men and their families (e.g. Ireland (193)), while others have a gender equality policy designed to involve men and boys (e.g. Sweden (194)). A deeper understanding of mental health-care reforms in post-Soviet countries is also needed, including the Russian Federation (195).

3.2.2 Shifting models of masculinity

In recent years, theory and research on men and masculinities have moved beyond an exclusively negative portrayal of masculinity as being damaging to men and their significant others towards gathering evidence of inclusive, caring and healthy masculinities. This shift was reflected in the reviewed literature. There was evidence that conformity to traditional masculinity norms, the impact of life events, and wider community and societal factors (e.g. prejudice, inequality and poverty) inhibit men from help-seeking. There were also examples of mens' efforts to resist the more unhelpful norms (e.g. difficulty in expressing emotions) and to incorporate softer elements into their masculine identities (e.g. displaying vulnerability), where circumstances allowed (privileged men with greater access to economic and cultural capital were better able to grow their masculinity). Men experiencing disadvantage, discrimination and social exclusion may lack the opportunities and support to develop healthier masculinities. Positive, progressive masculinities are increasingly being promoted across the media and popular culture, and this may persuade boys and young men to reject toxic masculinities in favour of personal, relational and social well-being.

However, some gender-sensitive interventions (116) are leveraging traditional norms to persuade men to seek help for mental health issues, for example by presenting help-seeking as requiring strength, independence and action and as protecting and enhancing valued masculine pursuits such as work, fatherhood and sporting activities.

3.2.3 Areas for further research

Despite a recent interest in male mental health issues, there is scope for further research; in particular, empirical research was notably lacking in the Russian literature (25). More research is also required to identify how men who have successfully engaged with mental health services have managed their masculinity concerns, with a view to identifying strategies most likely to be successful in specified contexts and for specific communities (50,106,107,112). In addition, promising community programmes designed to tackle men's mental health (including online initiatives) need to be independently evaluated to provide data on their effectiveness (75). It is also essential to track men who do not attend or drop out of therapy programmes in order to identify further barriers/facilitators and improve mental health promotion for all men.

More generally, there is a need to develop an interdisciplinary research programme on culture, men, gender, masculinities and mental health involving masculinity studies scholars, gender and social psychology specialists, and mental health practitioners across the WHO European Region. This should encompass local, regional and national studies using qualitative and quantitative intersectional methodologies. General principles and local community values derived from the resulting evidence base could be incorporated into tailored mental health programmes (incorporate project evaluations) for specific groups of men.

3.3 Policy considerations

Based on the findings of this scoping review, the main policy considerations to promote and protect men's and boys' mental health in the WHO European Region are to:

- support the mental health needs of the most vulnerable or at-risk groups (refugee and migrant, indigenous, sexual and ethnic minority men) by tackling the root causes of disconnection and isolation through addressing the links between gender and homophobia/racism;
- provide resources to enable parents and relevant institutions (e.g. schools or youth centres) to engage boys and young men (particularly those from minority and disadvantaged backgrounds) in critical discussions of gender norms, identities and relations and the links between gender, gender inequality, health and well-being;
- promote collaboration and partnerships between the health sector and community organizations working with diverse groups of men on a range of projects (e.g. cultivating responsible and involved fatherhood, violence prevention, addressing substance abuse);
- educate health- and social-care professionals about how gender influences how men present with mental health problems;
- develop male-friendly initiatives tailored to the values, customs and priorities of those groups of men most in need, and actively engage the target groups in developing such initiatives;
- promote strengths-based approaches to men's mental health that build on positive aspects of traditional masculinity and normalize mental health issues such as depression within diverse communities; and
- engage with health-focused television programmes and websites that provide relevant information and enable men to share their problems with and receive support from experts/peers, and promote online support forums to men in all Member States of the WHO European Region.

4. CONCLUSIONS

Traditional notions of masculinity can inhibit men from seeking help for psychological problems, with a stronger impact on men who experience socioeconomic disadvantage, discrimination or marginalization (e.g. men in sexual minority, refugee and migrant, rural and ethnic minority groups). Despite the barriers presented by male socialization, local cultural norms and wider societal forces, the evidence identified ways to facilitate men's help-seeking for mental health issues – and the help being offered to men. For example, a supportive environment in which help-seeking is normalized can encourage men to discuss their emotional issues and seek help. In another strategy, reframing help-seeking as a more masculine behaviour in mental health promotion interventions, or by men themselves, may lead more men to engage. Finally, questioning traditional constructions of masculinity can help men to come to terms with their vulnerability and encourage help-seeking. However, despite recent interest in male mental health issues, there is scope for further work. There is a clear need for masculinity studies scholars, gender experts, social psychology specialists and mental health practitioners in the WHO European Region to develop an interdisciplinary research programme on culture, men, masculinities and gender equality, masculinity and mental health. This should include local, regional and national studies using qualitative and quantitative intersectional methodologies with a focus on the differing public perceptions of mental illness and masculinities across different Member States. General principles and local community values derived from the resulting evidence base could be incorporated into tailored mental health programmes for specific groups of men within Region and beyond.

REFERENCES

1. Strategy on women's health and well-being in the WHO European Region. Copenhagen: WHO Regional Office for Europe; 2016 (http://www.euro.who.int/__data/assets/pdf_file/0003/333912/strategy-womens-health-en.pdf?ua=1, accessed 16 April 2020).

2. WHO Regional Committee for Europe resolution: EUR/RC66/R8 on a strategy on women's health and well-being in the WHO European Region. Copenhagen: WHO Regional Office for Europe; 2016 (http://www.euro.who.int/__data/assets/pdf_file/0020/319115/66rs08e_WomensHealth_160768.pdf?ua=1, accessed 16 April 2020).

3. WHO Regional Committee for Europe resolution EUR/RC68/R4 on a strategy on the health and well-being of men in the WHO European Region. Copenhagen: WHO Regional Office for Europe; 2018 (http://www.euro.who.int/__data/assets/pdf_file/0019/382240/68rs04e_MensHealthStrategy_180668.pdf?ua=1, accessed 16 April 2020).

4. Report of the 68th session of the WHO Regional Committee for Europe, Rome, 17–20 September 2018. Copenhagen: WHO Regional Office for Europe; 2018 (http://www.euro.who.int/__data/assets/pdf_file/0008/392507/68rp00e_Report_RC68_180641.pdf?ua=1, accessed 16 April 2020).

5. The health and well-being of men in the WHO European Region: better health through a gender approach. Copenhagen: WHO Regional Office for Europe; 2018 (http://www.euro.who.int/__data/assets/pdf_file/0007/380716/mhr-report-eng.pdf?ua=1, accessed 19 March 2020).

6. Transforming our world: the 2030 agenda for sustainable development. New York: United Nations; 2015 (General Assembly resolution 70/1; http://www.un.org/ga/search/view_doc.asp?symbol=A/RES/70/1&Lang=E, accessed 16 April 2020).

7. Health 2020: a European policy framework supporting action across government and society for health and well-being. Copenhagen: WHO Regional Office for Europe; 2013 (EUR/RC62/9; http://www.euro.who.int/__data/assets/pdf_file/0006/199536/Health2020-Short.pdf?ua=1, accessed 16 April 2020).

8. Sustainable Development Goals [website]. New York: United Nations; 2015 (https://sustainabledevelopment.un.org/?menu=1300, accessed 16 April 2020).

9. Gough B, Robertson S, editors. Men, masculinities and health: critical perspectives. Basingstoke: Palgrave MacMillan; 2010.

10. Oliffe JL, Han CSE, Ogrodniczuk JS, Phillips JC, Roy P. Suicide from the perspectives of older men who experience depression: a gender analysis. Am J Mens Health. 2011;5(5):444–54. doi: https://doi.org/10.1177/1557988311408410.

11. Шаповалов РА. Отношение мужчин к психологической помощи В кн.: Ежегодник по консультативной психологии, коучингу и консалтингу. Отв. ред.: В. Ю. Меновщиков,

А. Б. Орлов. Вып. 2. М. [Masculinity and the attitude of men to psychological assistance. In: Меновщиков ВЮ, Орлов АБ, editors. Yearbook of advisory psychology, coaching and consulting. Vol. 2]. Москва: Институт консультативной психологии и консалтинга (ФПК-Институт); 2015:63–72 (in Russian).

12. Пичиков АА, Попов ЮВ. "Гендерный парадокс" суицидального поведения [The "gender paradox" of suicidal behaviour]. Обозрения психиатрии и медицинской психологии им. В.М.Бехтерева. 2015;2:22–9 (in Russian).

13. Richards DA, Borglin G. Implementation of psychological therapies for anxiety and depression in routine practice: two-year prospective cohort study. J Affect Disord. 2011;133(1–2):51–60. doi: 10.1016/j.jad.2011.03.024.

14. Addis ME. Gender and depression in men. Clin Psychol Sci Pract. 2008;15(3):153–68. doi: 10.1111/j.1468-2850.2008.00125.x.

15. Гафаров ВВ, Громова ЕА, Гагулин ИВ, Панов ДО, Гафарова АВ. Гендерные особенности риска развития сердечно-сосудистых заболеваний у населения с симптомами депрессии в Сибири (программа ВОЗ "MONICA-PSYCHOSOCIAL") [Gender peculiarities of the risk of cardiovascular diseases in a population with symptoms of depression in Siberia (the WHO MONICA-psychosocial programme)]. Ter Arkh. 2017;89(9):60–7 (in Russian). doi: 10.17116/terarkh201789960-67.

16. Deverill C, King M. Common mental disorders. In: McManus S, Meltzer H, Brugha T, Bebbington P, Jenkins R, editors. Adult psychiatric morbidity in England, 2007. Results of a household survey. Leeds: NHS Health and Social Care Information Centre; 2009:25–52 (https://digital.nhs.uk/data-and-information/publications/statistical/adult-psychiatric-morbidity-survey/adult-psychiatric-morbidity-in-england-2007-results-of-a-household-survey, 23 March 2020).

17. Шатилова ЕС. Почему женщины подвержены депрессии гораздо чаще, чем мужчины? [Why are women more likely to be depressed than men?]. Академическая публицистика. 2018;9:111–16 (in Russian).

18. Разводовский ЮЕ. Алкогольные проблемы в России и Белоруссии: сравнительный анализ трендов [Alcohol problems in the Russian Federation and Belarus: a comparative analysis of trends]. Российский медико-биологический вестник им. Академика И.П. Павлова. 2017;25(2):237–46 (in Russian).

19. Roxburgh M, Donmall M, Wright C, Jones A. Statistics from the National Drug Treatment Monitoring System (NDTMS). 1 April 2010–31 March 2011. Vol. 1: the numbers. London: Department of Health/NHS National Treatment Agency for Substance Misuse; 2011 (https://www.drugsandalcohol.ie/16042/1/statisticsfromndtms201011vol1thenumbers%5B1%5D.pdf, accessed 19 March 2020).

20. Wilkins D. Untold problems: a review of the essential issues in the mental health of men and boys. London: Men's Health Forum; 2010 (https://www.bl.uk/collection-items/untold-problems-a-review-of-the-essential-issues-in-the-mental-health-of-men-and-boys#, accessed 19 March 2020).

21. Кузьминых АА, Ениколопов СН. Бытующие представления о мужской и женской агрессии [Prevailing ideas about male and female aggression]. Психологическая наука и образование. 2011;5:70–8 (in Russian).

22. Courtenay W. Constructions of masculinity and their influence on men's well-being: a theory of gender and health. Soc Sci Med. 2000;50(10):1385–401. doi: 10.1016/s0277-9536(99)00390-1.

23. Борискин МЛ, Улесикова ИВ, Шатыр ЮА, Мулик ИГ, Булатецкий СВ, Мулик ВБ. Возрастные и гендерные особенности предрасположенности человека к рискованному поведению [Age and gender traits of a person's predisposition to risky behaviour]. Личность в меняющемся мире: здоровье, адаптация, развитие. 2018;6:741–56 (in Russian).

24. Addis ME, Mahalik J. Men, masculinity and the contexts of help seeking. Am Psychol. 2003;58(1):5–14. doi: 10.1037/0003-066x.58.1.5.

25. Костенко МА. Психосоциальная помощь мужчинам трудоспособного возраста в контексте социально-демографической политики: контекст постановки проблемы [Psychosocial assistance to men of working age in the context of sociodemographic policy: statement on the context of the problem]. Социальная интеграция и развитие этнокультур в евразийском пространстве. 2013;1:153–7 (in Russian).

26. Carrigan T, Connell RW, Lee J. Toward a new sociology of masculinity. Theory Soc. 1985;14(5):551–604. doi: https://doi.org/10.1007/BF00160017.

27. Connell RW. Masculinities. Cambridge: Polity Press; 1995.

28. Connell RW, Messerschmidt JW. Hegemonic masculinity: rethinking the concept. Gend Soc. 2005;19(6):829–59. doi: https://doi.org/10.1177/0891243205278639.

29. Кон ИС. Гегемонная маскулинность как фактор мужского (не)здоровья [Hegemonic masculinity as a factor in male (non)health]. Социология: теория, методы, маркетинг: научно-теоретический журнал. 2008;4:5–16 (in Russian).

30. Кон ИС. Гендер и маскулинность, сыновья и отцы [Gender and masculinity, sons and fathers]. Журнал социологии и социальной антропологии. 2012;15(1):48–64 (in Russian).

31. Кон ИС. Мужчина в меняющемся мире [A man in a changing world]. Москва: Время; 2009 (in Russian).

32. Чернова ЖВ. "Корпоративный стандарт" современной мужественности. Инструкции по созданию [The "corporate standard" of modern masculinity. Instructions for construction]. Социологические исследования. 2003;2:97–104 (in Russian).

33. Тартаковская ИН. "Несостоявшаяся маскулинность" как тип поведения на рынке труда. Попкова ЛН, Тартаковская ИН. (ред.) Гендерные отношения в современной России: исследования 1990-х годов ["Failed masculinity" as a type of behaviour in the labour market. In: Попкова ЛН, Тартаковская ИН, editors. Gender relations in

the modern Russian Federation: 1990s studies]. Самара: Изд-во Самарского ун-та; 2003:42–70 (in Russian).

34. Тартаковская ИН. Смертельная ноша маскулинности [The fatal burden of masculinity]. Демоскоп Weekly. 2010;425–6 (in Russian).

35. Федосеева ИА. Опыт гендерного подхода в системе социального воспитания [An experience of the gender approach in the system of social education] [website]. Педагогические науки. 2012;2(12) (in Russian).

36. Connell RW. Masculinities, second edition. Cambridge: Polity Press; 2005.

37. Кон ИС. Мужская роль и гендерный порядок [Male role and gender order]. Вестник общественного мнения. 2008;2(94):37–43 (in Russian).

38. Хитрук ЕБ. "Мужской вопрос" в XXI в.: развитие комплексного подхода к изучению маскулинности ["Men's question" in the 21st century: the development of a comprehensive approach to the study of masculinity]. Женщина в российском обществе. 2016;2(79)91–7 (in Russian). doi: 10.21064/WinRS.2016.2.9.

39. Anderson E. Orthodox and inclusive masculinity: competing masculinities among heterosexual men in feminized terrain. Sociol Perspect. 2005;48(3):337–55. doi: https://doi.org/10.1525/sop.2005.48.3.337.

40. Bridges T, Pascoe CJ. Hybrid masculinities: new directions in the sociology of men and masculinities. Sociol Compass. 2014;8(3):246–58. doi: https://doi.org/10.1111/soc4.12134.

41. Atkinson M. Deconstructing men and masculinities. Toronto: Oxford University Press Canada; 2010 (Themes in Canadian Sociology).

42. MacDonald J. Building on the strength of Australian males. Int J Mens Health. 2011;10(1):82–96. doi: 10.3149/jmh.1001.82.

43. Sloan C, Gough B, Conner MT. Healthy masculinities? How ostensibly healthy men talk about lifestyle, health and gender. Psychol Health. 2010;25(7):783–803. doi: 10.1080/08870440902883204.

44. Hearn J, Pringle K. European perspectives on men and masculinities. Basingstoke: Palgrave; 2006.

45. Connell RW, Wood J. Globalization and business masculinities. Men Masc. 2005;7(4):347–64. doi: https://doi.org/10.1177/1097184X03260969.

46. Takakura H. The concept of manhood in post-socialist Siberia: the Sakha father as a wise hunter and a pastoralist. Sibirica. 2009;8:45–67. doi: https://doi.org/10.3167/sib.2009.080104.

47. Aimar V. Blurring masculinities in the Republic of Sakha, the Russian Federation. Polar Geogr (Palm Beach). 2018;41(2):1–19. doi: 10.1080/1088937X.2018.1498141.

48. Аннес А, Редлин М. Деревенская мужественность (маскулинность) [Rural manliness (masculinity)]. Ежегодник финно-угорских исследований. 2010;2:136–43 (in Russian).

49. Шаповалов РА. Опыт обращения за психологической помощью как фактор отношения мужчин к психотерапии [Experience of seeking psychological help as a factor in men's attitude to psychotherapy]. В кн.: Психология XXI века: российская психология в контексте мировой науки. Материалы международной научной конференции молодых ученых. СПб: Скифия-принт; 2016; 202–3 (in Russian).

50. Останин ИК, Тимохин ВВ. Отношение современных российских мужчин к обращению за профессиональной психологической помощью [Attitudes of contemporary Russian men to seeking professional psychological help]. В сборнике: Психология в современном мире сборник статей Международной научно-практической конференции. Кащеева ОВ, Антоненко ИВ, Карицкого ИН, редакторы. 2017; 382–3 (in Russian).

51. Богатушина ЯВ, Ковалева ЮЛ. Представления о психологической помощи в связи с субъективным запросом и личностными особенностями [Perceptions of psychological assistance as a result of an individual's request and specifics]. Правительство Санкт-Петербурга: Научные исследования выпускников факультета психологии Санкт-Петербургский государственный университет. 2016;4:32–8 (in Russian).

52. Хитрук ЕБ. Социально-психологическая поддержка мужчин в контексте "мужских проблем" [Psychosocial support for men in the context of "men's problems"]. Социологические исследования. 2017;11(403):122–8 (in Russian).

53. Розанов ВА. Самоубийства, психо-социальный стресс и потребление алкоголя в странах бывшего СССР [Suicide, psychosocial stress and alcohol consumption in the countries of the former USSR]. Суицидология. 2012;4:28–40 (in Russian).

54. Artazcoz L, Benach J, Borrell C, Cortès I. Unemployment and mental health: understanding the interactions. Am J Public Health. 2004;94(1):82–8. doi: 10.2105/ajph.94.1.82.

55. Antonakakis N, Collins A. The impact of fiscal austerity on suicide: on the empirics of a modern Greek tragedy. Soc Sci Med. 2014;112:39–50. doi: 10.1016/j.socscimed.2014.04.019.

56. Parkinson J, Minton J, Lewsey J, Bouttell J, McCartney G. Recent cohort effects in suicide in Scotland: a legacy of the 1980s? J Epidemiol Community Health. 2017;71(2):194–200. doi: 10.1136/jech-2016-207296.

57. Johnson JL, Oliffe JL, Kelly MT, Gladas P, Ogrodniczuk JS. Men's discourses of help-seeking in the context of depression. Sociol Health Illn. 2012;34(3):345–61. doi: 10.1111/j.1467-9566.2011.01372.x.

58. Шаповалов РА, Колпачников ВВ. Проблема отношения мужчин к психологической помощи [The problem of men's attitudes to psychological assistance]. Мир психологии: Научно-методический журнал. 2019;1(97):152–64 (in Russian).

59. Коломасова ЕН. Сущность и специфика социальных проблем мужчин в современном обществе [The nature and specificity of men's social problems in contemporary society]. Вестник Мордовского университета. 2010;2:172–6 (in Russian).

60. Sadler K, Bebbington P. Psychosis. In: McManus S, Meltzer H, Brugha T, Bebbington P, Jenkins R, editors. Adult psychiatric morbidity in England, 2007. Results of a household survey. Leeds: NHS Health and Social Care Information Centre; 2009:89–104 (https://digital.nhs.uk/data-and-information/publications/statistical/adult-psychiatric-morbidity-survey/adult-psychiatric-morbidity-in-england-2007-results-of-a-household-survey, accessed 19 March 2020).

61. Population in custody: monthly tables. March 2009: England and Wales. London: Ministry of Justice; 2009 (Statistics bulletin; https://assets.publishing.service.gov.uk/government/uploads/system/uploads/attachment_data/file/218179/population-in-custody-march-09.pdf, accessed 19 March 2020).

62. Озерова ОВ. Приверженность алкоголю в России: социальные различия и тенденции в 1990-е и 2000-е гг. [Alcohol dependence in the Russian Federation: social differences and trends in the 1990s and 2000s]. Журнал социологии и социальной антропологии. 2016;19(1):194–208 (in Russian).

63. O'Donnell S, Richardson N. Middle-aged men and suicide in Ireland. Dublin: Men's Health Forum in Ireland; 2018 (https://www.hse.ie/eng/services/publications/mentalhealth/middle-aged-men-and-suicide-in-ireland-executive-summary.pdf, accessed 19 March 2020).

64. Wyllie C, Platt S, Brownlie J, Chandler A, Connolly S, Evans R et al. Men, suicide and society: why disadvantaged men in mid-life die by suicide. Ewell: Samaritans; 2012 (Research report; https://media.samaritans.org/documents/Samaritans_MenSuicideSociety_ResearchReport2012.pdf, accessed 19 March 2020).

65. Key facts and trends in mental health: 2016 update. London: Mental Health Network, NHS Confederation; 2016 (Factsheet, March 2016; https://www.nhsconfed.org/-/media/Confederation/Files/Publications/Documents/MHN-key-facts-and-trends-factsheet_Fs1356_3_WEB.pdf?dl=1, accessed 19 March 2020).

66. Fazel S, Baillargeon J. The health of prisoners. Lancet. 2011;377(9769):956–65. doi: 10.1016/S0140-6736(10)61053-7.

67. Reeve K. The hidden truth about homelessness: experiences of single homelessness in England. London: Crisis; 2011 (Report summary, May 2011; https://www.crisis.org.uk/media/236816/the_hidden_truth_about_homelessness_es.pdf, accessed 19 March 2020).

68. Mahalik JR, Burns SM, Syzdek M. Masculinity and perceived normative health behaviors as predictors of men's health behaviors. Soc Sci Med. 2007; 64(11):2201–9. doi: 10.1016/j.socscimed.2007.02.035.

69. Рогачева ТВ. Влияние гендерных особенностей на здоровье [How gender affects health]. Сибирский психологический журнал. 2012:44;23-30 (in Russian).

70. Тулузакова МВ. Патриархальность и маскулинность как принцип организации гендерных отношений в российском обществе. [Patriarchy and masculinity as a principle of organizing gender relations in the Russian society]. Вестник Саратовского государственного технического университета. 2011;4(59):233–8 (in Russian).

71. Andersen I, Osler M, Petersen L, Grønbæk M, Prescott E. Income and risk of ischaemic heart disease in men and women in a Nordic welfare country. Int J Epidemiol. 2003;32:367–74. doi: 10.1093/ije/dyg073.

72. Kato-Wallace J, Barker G, Sharafi L, Mora L, Lauro G. Adolescent boys and young men: engaging them as supporters of gender equality and health and understanding their vulnerabilities. Washington (DC): Promundo US; 2016.

73. Hyde MK, Newton RU, Galvão DA, Gardiner RA, Occhipinti S, Lowe A et al. Men's help-seeking in the first year after diagnosis of localised prostate cancer. Eur J Cancer Care. 2017;26(2): e12497. doi: 10.1111/ecc.12497.

74. Robertson S, Gough B, Hanna E, Raine G, Robinson M, Seims A et al. Successful mental health promotion with men: evidence from "tacit knowledge". Health Prom Int. 2018;33(2):334–44. doi: 10.1093/heapro/daw067.

75. Рахлина ЕВ. Психологическая работа с мужчинами, применяющими насилие в близких отношениях. Опыт работы психолога Санкт-Петербургского государственного бюджетного учреждения "Центр социальной помощи семье и детям 'Аист' Пушкинского района" [Psychological work with men who use violence in close relationships. Experience of a psychologist of the Saint Petersburg publically funded organization "Stork" Centre for Social Assistance to Family and Children of the Pushkin District]. Социальное обслуживание семей и детей: научно- методический сборник. Вып. 11: Социальная работа с мужчинами. 2017;11:108–22 (in Russian).

76. Robertson S. Understanding men and health: masculinities, identity and well-being. Maidenhead: Open University Press; 2007.

77. Griffith D, Allen JO, Gunter K. Social and cultural factors influence African American men's medical help seeking. Res Soc Work Pract. 2011;21(3):337–47. doi: https://doi.org/10.1177/1049731510388669.

78. Темкина АА, Здравомыслова ЕА. Интерсекциональный поворот в гендерных исследованиях [Intersectional turn in gender studies]. Журнал социологии и социальной антропологии. 2017;20(5):15–38.

79. Robinson M, Keating F, Robertson S. Ethnicity, gender and mental health. Divers Equal Health Care. 2011;8(2):81–92.

80. Кузнецова ЛВ, Которский ВН, Торгашева ИВ. Психологическая диагностика в профилактике суицида у людей с гомосексуальной ориентацией. Бехтерев и

современная психология человечности. Сборник статей V Международной научно-практической конференции [Psychological diagnosis for suicide prevention among individuals with a homosexual orientation. In: Ankylosing spondylitis and modern psychology of humanity. Collection of articles of the V International scientific and practical conference]. Москва: Высшая Школа Экономики; 2015:454–66 (in Russian).

81. Guasp A. Gay and bisexual men's health survey (2013). London: Stonewall; 2015.

82. APA Working Group on Health Disparities in Boys and Men. Health disparities in racial/ethnic and sexual minority boys and men. Washington (DC): American Psychological Association; 2018 (Report; https://www.apa.org/pi/health-disparities/resources/race-sexuality-men-report.pdf, accessed 19 March 2020).

83. Griffith DM, Bruce MA, Thorpe RJ Jr, editors. Men's health equity: a handbook. New York: Routledge; 2019.

84. Hammer JH, Vogel DL. Men's help seeking for depression: the efficacy of a male-sensitive brochure about counseling. Couns Psychol. 2010;38(2):296–313. doi: 10.1177/0011000009351937.

85. Sierra Hernandez CA, Han C, Oliffe JL, Ogrodniczuk JS. Understanding help-seeking among depressed men. Psychol Men Masc. 2014;15(3):346–54. doi: http://dx.doi.org/10.1037/a0034052.

86. Levant RF, Stefanov DG, Rankin TJ, Halter MJ, Mellinger C, Williams CM. Moderated path analysis of the relationships between masculinity and men's attitudes toward seeking psychological help. J Couns Psychol. 2013;60(3):392–406. doi: 10.1037/a0033014.

87. Tedstone Doherty D, Kartalova-O'Doherty Y. Gender and self-reported mental health problems: predictors of help seeking from a general practitioner. Br J Health Psychol. 2010;15(1):213–28. doi: 10.1348/135910709X457423.

88. Yousaf O, Grunfield EA, Hunter MS. A systematic review of the factors associated with delays in medical and psychological help-seeking among men. Health Psychol Rev. 2015;9(2):264–76. doi: 10.1080/17437199.2013.840954.

89. O'Loughlin RE, Duberstein PR, Veazie PJ, Bell RA, Rochlen AB, Fernandez y Garcia E et al. Role of the gender-linked norm of toughness in the decision to engage in treatment for depression. Psychiatr Serv. 2011;62(7):740–6. doi: 10.1176/ps.62.7.pss6207_0740.

90. Call BS, Shafer K. Gendered manifestations of depression and help seeking among men. Am J Mens Health. 2018;12(1):41–51. doi: 10.1177/1557988315623993.

91. Herbst DM, Griffith NR, Slama KM. Rodeo cowboys: conforming to masculine norms and help-seeking behaviors for depression. J Rural Ment Health. 2014;38(1):20–35. doi: https://doi.org/10.1037/rmh0000008.

92. Harding C, Fox C. It's not about "Freudian couches and personality changing drugs": an investigation into men's mental health help-seeking enablers. Am J Mens Health. 2015;9(6):451–63. doi: 10.1177/1557988314550194.

93. Abraham T, Cheny AM, Curran GM. A Bourdieusian analysis of US military culture ground in the mental help-seeking literature. Am J Mens Health 2017;11(5):1358–65. doi: https://doi.org/10.1177/1557988315596037.

94. DeLenardo S, Lennox Terrion J. Suck it up: opinions and attitudes about mental illness stigma and help-seeking behaviour of male varsity football players. Can J Commun Ment Health. 2014;33(3):43–56. doi: https://doi.org/10.7870/cjcmh-2014-023.

95. Wirback T, Forsell Y, Larsson J.-O, Engström K, Edhborg M. Experiences of depression and help-seeking described by young Swedish men. Psychol Men Masc. 2018;19(3):407–17. doi: https://doi.org/10.1037/men0000110.

96. Tang M, Oliffe JL, Galdas PM, Phinney A, Han CS. College men's depression-related help-seeking: a gender analysis. J Ment Health. 2014;23(5):219–24. doi: 10.3109/09638237.2014.910639.

97. Berger JL, Addis ME, Green JD, Mackowiak C, Goldberg V. Men's reactions to mental health labels, forms of help-seeking, and sources of help-seeking advice. Psychol Men Masc. 2013;14(4):433–43. doi: https://doi.org/10.1037/a0030175.

98. Hoy S. Beyond men behaving badly: a meta-ethnography of men's perspectives on psychological distress and help seeking. Int J Mens Health. 2012;11(3):202–26. doi: 10.3149/jmh.1103.202.

99. Roy P, Tremblay G, Robertson S. Help-seeking among male farmers: connecting masculinities and mental health. Sociol Rural. 2014;54(4):460–76. doi: https://doi.org/10.1111/soru.12045.

100. Parent MC, Hammer JH, Bradstreet TC, Schwartz EN, Jobe T. Men's mental health help-seeking behaviors: an intersectional analysis. Am J Mens Health. 2018;12(1):64–73. doi: 10.1177/1557988315625776.

101. Seidler ZE, Dawes AJ, Rice SM, Oliffe JL Dhillon HM. The role of masculinity in men's help-seeking for depression: a systematic review. Clin Psychol Rev. 2016;49:106–18. doi: https://doi.org/10.1016/j.cpr.2016.09.002.

102. Ogrodniczuk JS, Oliffe JL, Black N. Canadian men's perspectives of depression: awareness and intention to seek help. Am J Mens Health. 2017;11(4):877–9. doi: 10.1177/1557988316669617.

103. Yousaf O, Popat A, Hunter MS. An investigation of masculinity attitudes, gender, and attitudes toward psychological help-seeking. Psychol Men Masc. 2015;16(2):234–37. doi: 10.1037/a0036241.

104. Pittius M. Man enough: the influence of masculinity scripts on help-seeking behaviors among men with depression [thesis]. Gothenburg: University of Gothenburg; 2014.

105. Gough B. Men's depression talk online: a qualitative analysis of accountability and authenticity in help-seeking and support formulations. Psychol Men Masc. 2016;17(2):156–64. doi: https://doi.org/10.1037/a0039456.

106. Датий АИ, Ганишина ИС, Кузнецова АС. Характеристика больных наркоманией осужденных мужчин, обратившихся за психологической помощью [Characteristics of drug addicted convicted men who sought psychological help]. Вестник Пермского института ФСИН России. 2014;2(13):21–5 (in Russian).

107. Датий АВ. Характеристика ВИЧ-инфицированных осужденных мужчин, обратившихся за психологической помощью [Characteristics of HIV-infected convicted men seeking psychological help]. Медицина. 2014;Т2,1(5):1–9 (in Russian).

108. Архиреева ТВ. Возможности психологического сопровождения становления ответственного отцовства Развитие детско-взрослых сообществ в условиях многообразия. Сборник статей по материалам Международной научно-практической конференции. Сост. ЕВ Иванов. [Opportunities for psychological support for the development of responsible fatherhood. In: Child–adult communities in a diverse environment. Collection of articles on the materials of the International scientific-practical conference, 24–25 April 2017. Compiled by EV Ivanov]. Великий Новгород: Новгородский государственный университет имени Ярослава Мудрого; 2017:149–64 (in Russian).

109. Платонова НМ (ред.). Семья и домашнее насилие. Практика консультирования мужчин – субъектов домашнего насилия Учебное пособие. 2-е изд, испр [Family and domestic violence – counselling practice for male subjects of domestic violence. Tutorial, second edition]. СанктПетербург: "Реноме"; 2014 (in Russian).

110. Меринов АВ, Меденцева ТА. Потенциальное желание обращения к специалисту в области психического здоровья у юношей: значение для суицидологической практики [Potential desire of young men to seek help from a mental health specialist: implications for suicidological practice]. Суицидология. 2016;7(2(23)):29–35 (in Russian).

111. Погудина ЕЮ. Деконструкция мифа о "настоящем мужчине" в практике психологического консультирования родителей. Комплексные исследования человека: психология: материалы VII Сибирского психологического форума. Ч. 1: Аттракторы и идентичности человека цифровой эпохи. Образование. Воспитание. Творчество [Deconstructing the myth of the "real man" in the practice of psychological counselling of parents. In: Integrated human research: psychology: materials of the VII Siberian Psychological Forum. Part 1: Attractors and human identities of the digital age. Education. Parenting. Creation]. Томск: Издательский Дом ТГУ; 2017:180–2 (in Russian).

112. Арпентьева МР. Трудные ситуации психотерапии и психологического консультирования подростков и юношей [Difficult situations of psychotherapy and psychological counselling of adolescents and boys]. В сборнике: Актуальные проблемы подростково-юношеской психиатрии Материалы Всероссийской научно-практической конференция с международным участием, посвященной памяти профессора М.Я. Цуцульковской. Москва: Научный центр психического здоровья; 2015:38–44 (in Russian).

113. Ковалева ЮЛ, Логинова НВ. Представления о психологическом консультировании у мужчин и женщин и профессиональный тип [Ideas about psychological counselling in men and women and professional type]. Сборники конференций НИЦ Социосфера. 2015;38:53–9 (in Russian).

114. Хижун НП. Опыт группового психологического консультирования мужчин с зависимыми формами поведения проекта "Дом на полдороги" в благотворительной организации "Ночлежка" [Experience of group psychological counselling of men with dependent forms of behavior in the project "Halfway house" of the Night-bed charity] Социальное обслуживание семей и детей: научно-методический сборник. 2017; 12:144–51 (in Russian).

115. Малышева АГ, Середа МВ. Редакторы. Научно-методический сборник "Социальное обслуживание семей и детей", Вып. 11, Социальная работа с мужчинами [Social work with men, Issue 1, Collection of research and methods articles "Social services to families and children"]. Санкт-Петербург: Городской информационно-методический центр "Семья", Правительство Санкт-Петербурга; 2017 (in Russian).

116. Gender mainstreaming for health managers: a practical approach. Participant's notes. Geneva: World Health Organization; 2011 (https://apps.who.int/iris/bitstream/handle/10665/44516/9789241501064_eng.pdf?sequence=2, accessed 18 April 2020).

117. Решетников ММ. Психическое здоровье населения – современные тенденции и старые проблемы [Mental health – current trends and old problems]. Национальный психологический журнал. 2015;1(17):9–15 (in Russian). doi: 10.11621/npj.2015.0102.

118. Березовская РА. Исследования отношения к здоровью: современное состояние проблемы в отечественной психологии [Research on attitudes to health: the current state of the problem in Russian psychology]. Вестник СПбГУ. 2011;12(1):221–6.

119. Shek O, Lumme-Sandt K, Pietilä I. Mental health care reforms in post-Soviet Russian media: negotiating new ideas and values. Eur J Mental Health. 2016;11(1–2):60–78. doi: https://doi.org/10.5708/EJMH.11.2016.1-2.4.

120. Diagnostic and statistical manual of mental disorders, fifth edition. Arlington (VA): American Psychiatric Association; 2013.

121. Pietilä I, Rytkönen M. "Health is not a man's domain": lay accounts of gender difference in life-expectancy in the Russian Federation. Soc Health Illn. 2008;30(7):1070–85. doi: 10.1111/j.1467-9566.2008.01106.x.

122. King M, Semlyen J, Tai SS, Killaspy H, Osborn D, Popelyuk D et al. A systematic review of mental disorder, suicide, and deliberate self-harm in lesbian, gay and bisexual people. BMC Psychiatry. 2008;8:70. doi: 10.1186/1471-244X-8-70.

123. Bahrke MS, Yesalis CE. Abuse of anabolic androgenic steroids and related substances in sport and exercise. Curr Opin Pharmacol. 2004;4(6):614–20. doi: 10.1016/j.coph.2004.05.006.

124. Moos RH, Schutte KK, Brennan PL, Moos BS. Older adults' alcohol consumption and late-life drinking problems: a 20-year perspective. Addiction. 2009;104(8):1293–302. doi: 10.1111/j.1360-0443.2009.02604.x.

125. Good GE, Wood PK. Male gender role conflict, depression, and help seeking: do college men face double jeopardy? J Couns Dev. 1995;74(1):70–5. doi 10.1002/j.1556-6676.1995.tb01825.x.

126. Ичитовкина ЕГ, Злоказова МВ, Соловьев АГ, Эпштейн АМ. Комплексная терапия психогенных расстройств комбатантов [Comprehensive therapy for psychogenic disorders of combatants]. Вестник современной клинической медицины. 2015;8(6):17–24 (in Russian).

127. Richardson LK, Frueh BC, Acierno R. Prevalence estimates of combat-related post-traumatic stress disorder: critical review. Aust N Z J Psychiatry. 2010;44(1):4–19. doi: 10.3109/00048670903393597.

128. Bryant-Davis T. Healing requires recognition: the case for race-based traumatic stress. Couns Psychol. 2007;35:135–42. doi: https://doi.org/10.1177/0011000006295152.

129. Вишняков АИ, Пашина АЮ. Гендерные особенности проявления синдрома эмоционального выгорания у сотрудников пожарной службы [Gender features of the manifestation of burnout syndrome among firefighters]. АНИ: педагогика и психология. 2016;5,4(17):314–16.

130. Hanna E, Gough B, Markham S. Masculinities in the construction industry: a double-edged sword for health and well-being? Gend Work Organ. 2020 (Epub ahead of print). doi: https://doi.org/10.1111/gwao.12429.

131. Milnes K, Turner-Moore T, Gough B, Denison J, Gatere L, Haslam C et al. Sexual bullying in young people across five European countries: summary research report for the Addressing Sexual Bullying Across Europe (ASBAE) project. Leeds: Leeds Beckett University; 2015.

132. Carrera-Fernández MV, Lameiras-Fernández M, Rodríguez-Castro Y. Performing intelligible genders through violence: bullying as gender practice and heteronormative control. Gend Educ. 2018;30(3):341–59. doi: https://doi.org/10.1080/09540253.2016.1203884.

133. Rivers I, Chesney T, Coyne IJ. Cyber-bullying. In: Monks CP, Coyne IJ, editors. Bullying in different contexts. Cambridge: Cambridge University Press; 2011:211–30.

134. Pascoe CJ. Notes on a sociology of bullying: young men's homophobia as gender socialization. QED: J GLBTQ Worldmaking. 2013;1:87–104. doi: 10.1353/qed.2013.0013.

135. Keating F. African and Caribbean men and mental health. Ethn Inequal Health Soc Care. 2009;2(2):41–53. doi: https://doi.org/10.1108/17570980200900015.

136. Глендиннинг Э, Попков ЮВ, Селезнева ЕВ. Ментальное здоровье современных подростков (по результатам социологического исследования в Республике

Алтай) [Mental health of modern teenagers (based on a sociological survey in the Altai Republic)]. Уральский исторический вестник. 2017;54(1):83–91 (in Russian).

137. Жигинас НВ. Проблемы психического здоровья и гендерной идентичности в подростковом возрасте [Challenges of mental health and gender identity at adolescence]. Вестник Томского государственного педагогического университета. 2015;3(156):85–9 (in Russian).

138. Абрамова МО, Сухушина ЕВ, Рыкун АЮ. Воспроизводство маскулинности: семья как основной агент социализации [Reproduction of masculinity: family as the main socialization agent]. Вестник Томского государственного университета Философия. Социология. Политология. 2018;41:80–9. doi: 10.17223/1998863X/41/10.

139. Priebe S, Giacco D, El-Nagib R. Public health aspects of mental health among migrants and refugees: a review of the evidence on mental health care for refugees, asylum seekers and irregular migrants in the WHO European Region. Copenhagen: WHO Regional Office for Europe; 2016 (Health Evidence Network (HEN) Synthesis Report 47; http://www.euro.who.int/__data/assets/pdf_file/0003/317622/HEN-synthesis-report-47.pdf?ua=1, accessed 19 March 2020).

140. Якимов АН. "В последний момент, на всякий случай, при крайней необходимости": проблемы и особенности социально-правовой поддержки мужчин – трудовых мигрантов ["At the last moment, just in case, in case of emergency": problems and features of sociolegal support for male labour migrants]. Социальное обслуживание семей и детей: научно-методический сборник. 2017;11:142–52 (in Russian).

141. Журавлева ИВ, Иванова ЛЮ. Мигранты: социально-экономические условия жизни, влияющие на здоровье, и обращаемость в российские медицинские учреждения (результаты опроса в Санкт-Петербурге) [Migrants: socioeconomic living conditions that affect health and access to Russian medical institutions (results of a survey in Saint Petersburg)]. Электронный научный журнал Социальные аспекты здоровья населения; 2015 (in Russian).

142. Ковешников АА. Культуральные факторы в генезе формирования алкогользависимового поведения [Cultural factors in the genesis of alcohol-dependent behaviour]. Вестник угроведения. 2015;3(22):119–28 (in Russian).

143. ProMundo's annual report 2015. Rio de Janeiro: ProMundo; 2015 (https://promundoglobal.org/wp-content/uploads/2016/08/Promundo-Annual-Report-2015-Final.pdf, accessed 19 March 2020).

144. Ashe F. The new politics of masculinity: men, power and resistance. Abingdon: Routledge; 2007.

145. Vandello JA, Bosson JK. Hard won and easily lost: a review and synthesis of theory and research on precarious manhood. Psychol Men Masc. 2013;14(2):101–13. doi: https://doi.org/10.1037/a0029386.

146. Kosakowska-Berezecka N, Besta T, Adamska K, Jaśkiewicz M, Jurek P, Vandello J. If my masculinity is threatened I won't support gender equality? The role of agentic self-stereotyping in restoration of manhood and perception of gender relations. Psychol Men Masc. 2016;17(3):274–84. doi: https://doi.org/10.1037/men0000016.

147. Dolan A. "You can't ask for a Dubonnet and lemonade!": working class masculinity and men's health practices. Sociol Health Illn. 2011;33(4):586–601. doi: 10.1111/j.1467-9566.2010.01300.x.

148. CALM [website]. London: Campaign Against Living Miserably; 2020 (https://www.thecalmzone.net, accessed 19 March 2020).

149. deVisser RO, Smith JA, McDonnell EJ. "That's not masculine": masculine capital and health-related behaviour. J Health Psychol. 2009;14(7):1047–58. doi: 10.1177/1359105309342299.

150. MacLean A, Sweeting H, Walker L, Patterson C, Räisänen U, Hunt K. "It's not healthy and it's decidedly not masculine": a media analysis of United Kingdom newspaper representations of eating disorders in males. BMJ Open. 2015;5(5):e007468. doi: 10.1136/bmjopen-2014-007468.

151. Men get eating disorders too [website]. Brighton: Mind in Brighton and Hove; 2020 (https://www.mindcharity.co.uk/the-mind-directory/men-get-eating-disorders-too/, accessed 17 April 2020).

152. Seymour-Smith S. A reconsideration of the gendered mechanisms of support in online interactions about testicular implants: a discursive approach. Health Psychol. 2013;32(1):91–9. doi: 10.1037/a0029507.

153. Hanna E, Gough B. Emoting infertility online: a qualitative analysis of men's forum posts. Health (Lond). 2016;20(4):363–82. doi: 10.1177/1363459316649765.

154. Bennet E, Gough B. In pursuit of leanness: the management of appearance, affect and masculinities within a men's weight management forum. Health. 2013;17(3):284–99. doi: 10.1177/1363459312454149.

155. Lowe A, Gough B. Homophobia, gender and sporting culture. Bristol: Sport Allies; 2016 (https://static1.squarespace.com/static/57ace591e58c628508b127f6/t/5c98ac4ca4222ff8226f7349/1553509641437/Sport%2BAllies%2BLeeds%2BBeckett%2BHomophobia%2BGender%2BSporting%2BCulture%2BReport%281%29.pdf, accessed 22 March 2020).

156. Who we are. Our mission. In: United Kingdom Men's Sheds Association [website]. Bristol: United Kingdom Men's Sheds Association; 2020 (https://menssheds.org.uk, accessed 19 March 2020).

157. Краевой кризисный центр для мужчин [Regional Crisis Centre for Men] [website]. Barnaul: Ministry of Social Protection of the Altai Region; 2020 (http://www.criscentr.ru, accessed 19 March 2020).

158. Кризисный центр для мужчин, пострадавших от насилия "Двоеточие" [The St Petersburg Centre for Men as Victims of Violence] [website]. Санкт-Петербург; 2020 (https://centerformen.ru, accessed 19 March 2020).

159. [State budgetary institution of the Komi Republic "Centre for the social rehabilitation of homeless, unemployed persons in Syktyvkar"] [website]. Сыктывкар: Государственное бюджетное учреждение Республики Коми "Центр социальной адаптации для лиц без определенного места жительства и занятий г.Сыктывкара"; 2020 (http://kcmsyktyvkar.rkomi.ru, accessed 1 May 2020).

160. Gray CM, Hunt K, Mutrie N, Anderson AS, Leishman J, Dalgarno L et al. Football fans in training: the development and optimization of an intervention delivered through professional sports clubs to help men lose weight, become more active and adopt healthier eating habits. BMC Public Health. 2013;13:232. doi: 10.1186/1471-2458-13-232.

161. Caddick N, Smith B, Phoenix C. The effects of surfing and the natural environment on the well-being of combat veterans. Qual Health Res. 2015;25:76–86. doi: 10.1177/1049732314549477.

162. Khaki M. Muslim men face pressure to ignore their mental health problems: it is time to stop the denial. In: Independent Voices. 15 June 2019 (https://www.independent.co.uk/voices/muslim-men-depression-mental-health-nationals-mens-health-week-a8960001.html, accessed 19 March 2020).

163. Male mental health. In: Taraki [website]. Taraki Well-being; 2020 (http://www.taraki.uk/male-mental-health, accessed 19 March 2020).

164. PSHE Association [website]. London: Personal Social and Health Education Association; 2020 (https://www.pshe-association.org.uk, accessed 19 March 2020).

165. Gunnell KE, Flament MF, Buchholz A, Henderson KA, Obeid N, Schubert N et al. Examining the bidirectional relationship between physical activity, screen time, and symptoms of anxiety and depression over time during adolescence. Prev Med. 2016;88:147–52. doi: 10.1016/j.ypmed.2016.04.002.

166. Good Lad Initiative: promoting positive masculinity [website]. Oxford: Good Lad Initiative; 2017 (https://www.goodladinitiative.com, accessed 17 February 2020).

167. ASBAE (Addressing Sexual Bullying Across Europe). In: DAPHNE toolkit [website]. Luxembourg: European Commission; 2020 (https://ec.europa.eu/justice/grants/results/daphne-toolkit/content/asbae-addressing-sexual-bullying-across-europe_en, accessed 19 March 2020).

168. Violence prevention: the evidence. Geneva: World Health Organization; 2010 (Series of briefings on violence prevention; https://www.who.int/violence_injury_prevention/violence/4th_milestones_meeting/evidence_briefings_all.pdf, accessed 19 March 2020).

169. Голованова НА. Проблемы борьбы с буллингом: законодательное решение [Challenges to combat bullying: a legislative solution]. Журнал российского права. 2018;8:113–23 (in Russian). doi: 10.12737/art_2018_8_11.

170. [Federal Resource Center for Psychological Services in the Education System] [website]. Москва; Федеральный ресурсный центр психологической службы в системе образования; 2020 (in Russian, http://www.frcp.ru, accessed 1 May 2020).

171. Health 2020: education and health through the life-course. Copenhagen: WHO Regional Office for Europe; 2015 (http://www.euro.who.int/__data/assets/pdf_file/0007/324619/Health-2020-Education-and-health-through-the-life-course-en.pdf?ua=1, accessed 19 March 2020).

172. Sasson I. Trends in life expectancy and lifespan variation by educational attainment: United States, 1990–2010. Demography. 2016;53(2):269–93. doi: 10.1007/s13524-015-0453-7.

173. Fortin NM, Oreopoulos P, Phipps S. Leaving boys behind: gender disparities in high academic achievement. J Hum Resour. 2015;50:549–79. doi: 10.3368/jhr.50.3.549.

174. Share of youth not in education, employment or training, male (% of male youth population). In: International Labour Organization ILOSTAT database [online database]. Washington (DC): World Bank; 2017 (https://data.worldbank.org/indicator/SL.UEM.NEET.MA.ZS, accessed 19 March 2020).

175. Report on discrimination of Roma children in education. Brussels: European Commission; 2014 (https://tandis.odihr.pl/bitstream/20.500.12389/21933/1/08101.pdf, accessed 19 March 2020).

176. Promundo, United Nations Population Fund, MenEngage. Engaging men and boys in gender equality and health: a global toolkit for action. New York: United Nations Population Fund; 2018 (https://www.unfpa.org/sites/default/files/pub-pdf/Engaging%20Men%20and%20Boys%20in%20Gender%20Equality.pdf, accessed 19 March 2020).

177. Клецина ИС, Чикалова ЕА. Взаимосвязь норм маскулинности и социальных представлений о содержании поведения в рамках отцовской роли [Relationship between masculinity norms and social perceptions of paternal behaviour]. Вестник Ленинградского государственного университета имени А.С.Пушкина. 2013; 2(5, Психология):24–35 (in Russian).

178. Bell J, Pustułka P. Multiple masculinities of Polish migrant men. NORMA. 2017;(2):127–43. doi: 10.1080/18902138.2017.1341677.

179. Греков ИМ, Шуменко МА. Ценностно-нормативные основы этнической культуры северокавказских народов и проблема особенностей этнической миграции на Юге России [The normative and value foundations of north Caucasian ethnic cultures and the problem of ethnic migration in southern the Russian Federation]. Гуманитарные и социально-экономические науки. 2014;4(77):46–51 (in Russian).

180. Stoeckl K. The Russian Orthodox Church as moral norm entrepreneur. Relig State Soc. 2016;44(2):132–51. doi: 10.1080/09637494.2016.1194010.

181. Wenger LM. Beyond ballistics: expanding our conceptualization of men's health-related help seeking. Am J Mens Health. 2011;5(6):488–99. doi: 10.1177/1557988311409022.

182. Martin LA, Neighbors HW, Griffith DM. The experience of symptoms of depression in men vs women: analysis of the National Comorbidity Survey Replication. JAMA Psychiatry. 2013;70(10):1100–6. doi: 10.1001/jamapsychiatry.2013.1985.

183. Кабышева ЭВ Образ "пацана" как выражение традиционных маскулинных черт в российском кино: характерные черты и причины актуальности [The image of a "boy" as an expression of traditional masculinity in Russian cinema: characteristic features and reasons for relevance]. Вестник Томского государственного университета. Культурология и искусствоведение; 2018;31:56–64.

184. Бычкова ОИ Герой нашего времени: ценности в зеркале российского телесериала [The hero of our times: values in the mirror of Russian television series]. Наследие веков. 2016;1:48–53.

185. Peretz T, Lehrer J, Dworkin SL. Impacts of men's gender-transformative personal narratives: a qualitative evaluation of the men's story project. Men Masc. 2020;23(1):104–26. doi: https://doi.org/10.1177/1097184X18780945.

186. Webb R. How not to be a boy. Edinburgh: Canongate Books; 2017.

187. All man: Grayson Perry on masculinity [documentary]. Channel 4, United Kingdom; 2016.

188. Gillette [website]. Cincinnati (OH): Procter & Gamble; 2020 (https://gillette.com/en-us/our-committment, accessed 19 March 2020).

189. In depth. What makes a man? In: Lynx [website]. London: Unilever; 2020 (https://www.lynxformen.com/uk/inspiration/culture/men-in-progress-1.html, accessed 19 March 2020).

190. БУЛАГ – Святой источник [Bulag – the sacred spring]. Лыгденов С, директор. Улан-Удэ: МонУла филмз; 2013 in Russian).

191. Завод [The factory]. Быков Ю, директор. Москва: Центральное партнерство; 2018.

192. Петрова ЕВ. Теоретическое исследование факторов отношения родителей к взрослым детям с гомо-/бисексуальной идентичностью [Theoretical study of factors of parents' attitude to adult children with homo/bisexual identity] [online publication]. Ученые записки: электронный научный журнал Курского государственного университета. 2015;1(33).

193. Department of Health, National Steering Committee, International Year of the Child, Healthy Ireland. National men's health action plan. Healthy Ireland – men: HI-M 2017–2021. Dublin: Department of Health; 2016 (https://www.lenus.ie/bitstream/handle/10147/621003/HealthyIrelandMen.pdf?sequence=1&isAllowed=y, accessed 19 March 2020).

194. Power, goals and agency: a feminist policy for a gender-equal future. Stockholm: Government Offices of Sweden; 2016 (Govt Comm 2016/17:10 summary; https://www.government.se/49c90f/globalassets/government/dokument/socialdepartementet/fact-sheet-summary-of-the-government-communication–power-goals-and-agency–a-feminist-policy, accessed 22 March 2020).

195. Shek O. Mental health care reforms in post-Soviet Russian Federation: negotiating new ideas and values [thesis]. Tampere: University of Tampere; 2018 (https://pdfs.semanticscholar.org/12f7/7a0be70a95f5f4b1f4b0c67c201eda1cab1a.pdf, accessed 19 March 2020).

ANNEX 1. SEARCH STRATEGY

Databases and websites

Searches were performed during March 2019 and there were no geographical limitations. The following databases were searched for peer-reviewed publications in English and in Russian using defined search terms: CINAHL (Cumulative Index to Nursing and Allied Health Literature), Project MUSE, PubMed, Scopus and Web of Science. As the search in Russian produced few relevant results, the search was expanded to include key Russian language databases: CyberLeninka, elibrary.RU, National Electronic Library, Google Academy (in Russian), the General Digital Catalogue of the Russian State Library and Scholar.ru, plus databases of selected university libraries (Lomonosov Moscow State University, Higher School of Economics, St Petersburg University). Internet searches of grey literature in English and in Russian were conducted in Ethos, Google and OpenGrey.

Search terms

Searches used four key search term categories, with all combinations of search terms (in English or Russian) used across all four categories:

1. men OR masculinity OR male OR gender
2. help-seeking OR engagement OR service use
3. mental health OR depression
4. culture.

Selection strategy

The same selection strategy was used for academic and grey literature. Advanced searches for keywords in only/both the title and abstract were used to ensure that only the most relevant results were found. Reference lists of recent relevant review papers were also checked to identify other suitable articles.

Inclusion criteria were:

- a primary focus on common mental health problems
- an analytic focus on masculinity
- a primary focus on help-seeking.

Exclusion criteria for titles and abstracts were a primary focus on:

- physical rather than mental health
- women
- symptoms, coping and treatment (with no reference to help-seeking).

Additional exclusion criteria for full-text articles were:

- a primary focus on severe mental health problems (i.e. psychosis)
- no or limited focus on masculinity.

For publications in English, of the initial 3197 titles and abstracts screened after removal of duplicates, full-text review was carried out for 155. Application of the additional exclusion criteria resulted in a set of 23 papers in English. For publications in Russian, a total of 399 titles and abstracts were screened after removal of duplicates, of which 124 were included in a full-text review, yielding a set 18 articles in Russian. A final set of 41 articles were included in the scoping review.

Further research papers, reports and policy documents were considered based on feedback from panel members attending the fifth WHO expert group meeting on the cultural contexts of health and well-being.

Initial separate scoping reviews of English and Russian publications using a methodology informed by the framework set out by Arksey and O'Malley (1), with adaptations by Levac, Colquhoun and O'Brien (2), were combined in the final review. The analysis was informed by feedback from expert reviewers on the first draft report.

Figs A1.1 and A1.2 illustrate the selection of studies in English and Russian, respectively, based on the PRISMA statement (3).

Fig. A1.1. Selection of studies in English

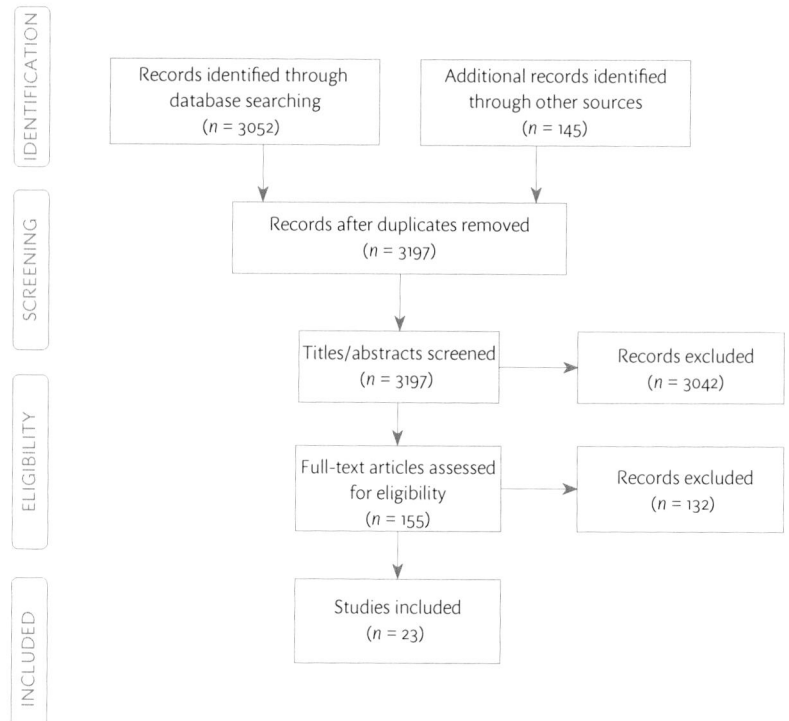

Fig. A1.2. Selection of studies in Russian

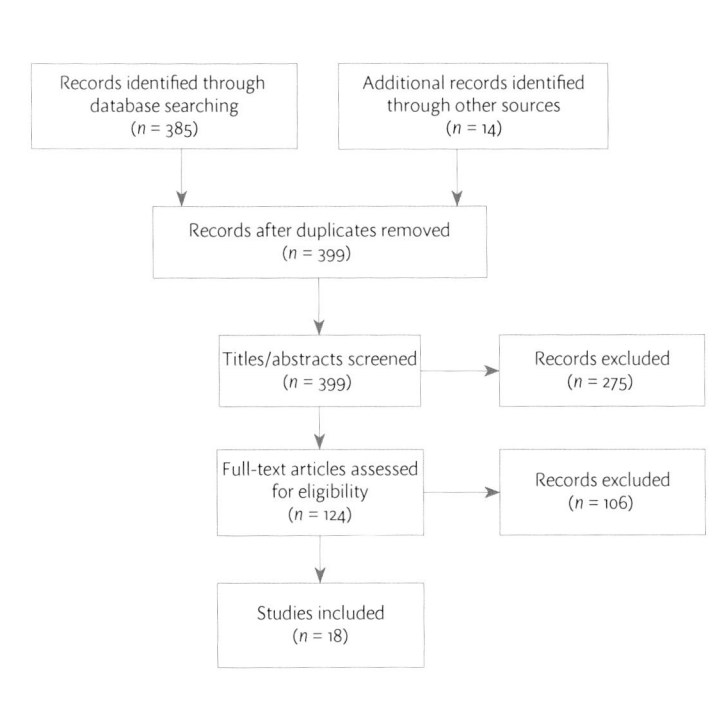

References

1. Arksey H, O'Malley L. Scoping studies: towards a methodological framework. Int J Soc Res Methodol. 2005;8(1):19–32. doi: 10.1080/1364557032000119616.

2. Levac D, Colquhoun H, O'Brien KK. Scoping studies: advancing the methodology. Implement Sci. 2010;5(1):1–9. doi: 10.1186/1748-5908-5-69.

3. Moher D, Liberati A, Tetzlaff J, Altman DG, PRISMA Group. Preferred reporting items for systematic reviews and meta-analyses: the PRISMA statement. PLOS Med. 2009;6(7):e1000097. doi: 10.1371/journal.pmed.1000097.